For ~~[scribbled]~~

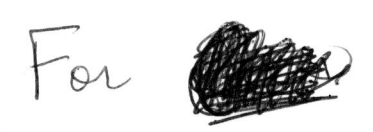

August 2022

FOREVER Grateful

Enjoy!

A TALE OF PERSEVERANCE

MELODY KLASSEN

Melody Klassen

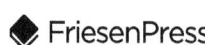
FriesenPress

One Printers Way
Altona, MB R0G 0B0
Canada

www.friesenpress.com

Copyright © 2022 by Melody Klassen
First Edition — 2022

All rights reserved.

No part of this publication may be reproduced in any form, or by any means, electronic or mechanical, including photocopying, recording, or any information browsing, storage, or retrieval system, without permission in writing from FriesenPress.

ISBN
978-1-03-913294-8 (Hardcover)
978-1-03-913293-1 (Paperback)
978-1-03-913295-5 (eBook)

1. BIOGRAPHY & AUTOBIOGRAPHY, PERSONAL MEMOIRS

Distributed to the trade by The Ingram Book Company

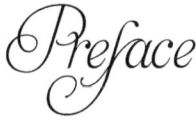

Preface

This book is my life according to me.
This is MY TRUTH.
I wrote this book with as much courage and clarity as possible.
I wrote these words for the purpose of
"show don't tell."
I wanted to show the power of gratitude and love.

Fill the earth with your songs of gratitude.
　　　　　—Charles Spurgeon

*Everything we do should be a result of our gratitude
for what God has done for us.*
　　　　　—Lauryn Hill

Dedication

This work of love is dedicated to all Canadians waiting for an organ and/or tissue transplant. May my words offer hope and strength.
Know that there is life after transplant.
To donors everywhere: thank you for your wonderful gifts. Whether you were a living donor or you've suffered the loss of a loved one, your "gift of life" has saved lives and made life better for all of us.
Again, thank you.
Finally, to my beautiful children: you've filled my life with love, happiness, and grandchildren.

Table of Contents

Preface .... *iii*
Dedication .... *vii*

Chapter 1
Call Me Melody/Daughter/Mom/Sister/Granny *1*

Chapter 2
Music Is in the Marrow of My Bones *7*

Chapter 3
School and Sick Notes *11*

Chapter 4
Keys to Creativity and Confidence *19*

Chapter 5
From the Mountains to the Valley *29*

Chapter 6
Wounded with Wisdom *43*

Chapter 7
In My Heart: David, Jay and Tim *55*

Chapter 8
In My Belly: Lauren *63*

Chapter 9
In My Life: My Kids Are My Joy *71*

Chapter 10
Lessons from Little Ones *75*

Chapter 11
Role Model *79*

Chapter 12
Summer from Hell 89

Chapter 13
Games: Me? An Athlete?. 101

Chapter 14
Unbelievable: Grandkids 113

Chapter 15
Grand Parenthood: What Fun 121

Chapter 16
Urgent Care, Good Care 129

Chapter 17
Dialysis, Drugs... or Death 135

Chapter 18
A Shocking Event 143

Chapter 19
Stroke of Insight 149

Chapter 20
A Week in My Life, Honest 157

Chapter 21
Where Am I Now?. 159

Chapter 22
Wanting the Last Word: COVID-19 163

Chapter 23
Looking Back, Looking Forward 175

Acknowledgements 183

Chapter 1

Call Me Melody/Daughter/Mom/Sister/Granny

When I tell people I was born in Saskatchewan, they always want to know where. This seems to be a pretty standard question for people to ask. Most people know little or nothing about Saskatchewan yet they initially claim to be interested in Canada's flattest province. When I tell them I was born in Moose Jaw, the Prairie's third largest "city" (pop: 32 000), the conversation usually ends there. Most people underestimate Saskatchewan and judge it as a boring place. They imagine flatness in every direction for miles and miles. For me, Saskatchewan is beautiful. For instance, the sky is so big it seems endless and you can enjoy varying colours: during the day, a calm, beautiful blue; and as the sun sets, shades of pink and orange.

Part of the largeness of the sky is because there are so few tall buildings in Saskatchewan. The aurora borealis (northern lights) can shine spectacularly all across Saskatchewan, showcasing blue, red, yellow, and green.

Although I have not been to Moose Jaw in many years, the city has come into its own by promoting its mysterious underground tunnels, attributed to Al Capone and his infamous bootlegging.

Like the tunnels in Moose Jaw, plenty of mystery remains around my lifelong health issues and why there were such long, dark stretches of pain and disappointment. From an early age I suffered from something that had no diagnosis, therefore could not be named or tamed. According to Western medicine, if an illness can't be defined, the illness doesn't exist, or worse: the sickness is inside your head. Mystery in life can feel exciting and make us feel grateful to be alive while inspiring a sense of adventure and wonder; we don't know what's going to happen next. But when your health is a source of mystery, meaning it's a mystery why you feel as terrible as you do, there is no excitement or joy. There's a sense you are fighting for your life and in a lot of cases, you are. You're not just fighting for your physical life but for your quality of life too.

I probably would have done better approaching my frail health and exasperated medical team more like an aggressive gangster than a polite little girl. My precarious health has shaped my life into patterns of ups and downs that border on criminal. Happily, I always knew justice would be served at some point. As I approach my seventh decade and feel comfortable looking back and forward, I see a tunnel of discovery that has travelled great distances in the dark but ultimately led me, and my beautiful family, above ground and into the light of well-being and grace.

When I was three years old and my health was perfectly fine, my family left Moose Jaw. My dad, a minister, received an opportunity to lead a church in Peterborough, Ontario. This was our very first family foray away from the west. What might have happened if we had stayed in Moose Jaw? Would my health have been as bad as it ended up being? Would I have been better cared for in a smaller town? Or would my decline have happened sooner? These are questions I admit that I sometimes indulge in on particularly tough physical days when energy and mood are low. There are no answers.

Chances are that staying in Moose Jaw would not have been the best scenario for my health, assuming my physical decline was destined irrespective of where I lived. Rural Saskatchewan, and in fact the entire province, simply did not have the medical resources available in southern Ontario. We moved to Peterborough. My health did what it did. And here is how life for me came to be.

I was born July 11th, 1956, to Ina and Wesley Klassen. Their three boys preceded me: David, Timothy, and James. Dad was a teacher and minister, which made me a "P.K.," a preacher's kid. Mom was, as most moms were at that time, a stay-at-home mom. When I was born my dad said to my brothers, "Each of you has a sister." It was a true statement but perhaps a bit confusing.

My oldest brother, David, was almost 10 years older than I and he did his best to make sure I did not get spoiled. David and I were not close until adulthood. One vivid example of our childhood dynamics was when I was in my late teens and our paternal grandmother visited from Manitoba. Having my grandmother there always added a layer of uneasiness. Our parents expected us to be on our best behaviour. Grandma did not come to visit often so it was a big deal to have her among us.

David started in on me, teasing and goading me about anything that pushed my buttons. It is so long ago that I cannot remember exactly what he was on about, but I do remember making a silent resolution: do not back down. My resolve just kept him going. Finally, Mom intervened (unfairly, in my opinion, since she told me to "let it go") and the teasing round with David came to an end. Of course, and as usual, I ended up in tears.

I was so upset with myself because I had violated my own decision to not back down or give up. Or cry. Throughout my childhood, and especially as I matured and came into my own, it was always hard standing up for myself. Wanting not to be teased, but to be cherished, by David and my other brothers was an ongoing battle of wits and whining.

My brother Tim, seven years older than I, was my hero. Every morning my mom would French braid my hair and I would cry. The tears were caused by Mom brushing out my hair and pulling each strand tight. Tim would do his best to distract me, always wanting to inspire a smile or giggle. At night if I had a bad dream or couldn't sleep, I knew I could crawl into bed with Tim and fall asleep immediately.

I guess it is no surprise that Tim, my favourite big brother, became my first kidney donor.

When my big brother Jay came along, the family was surprised. Mom had been convinced she was carrying a girl but I was not set to arrive for another four years. Jay and I were both cursed with the "youngest" label. Jay was the youngest boy and I was the youngest (and only) girl. Yet we did not share much else in common until we were older and more confident about our place in the family.

Like David, Jay believed he needed to ensure I did not get too spoiled. Like his two older brothers, Jay thought teasing me was a good way to make me humble and know my place in the household pecking order. Fodder for teasing me was limitless and if I cried, so much the better. I'm sure my parents were delighted to have so much help raising me!

My unusual (and very musical) name was chosen from a Billy Graham movie. At the time my parents lived in Moose Jaw, and their circle of friends consisted of three couples blessed with sons but few daughters. The group's favourite movie, "Oiltown U.S.A.," featured a heroine called Melody. The unusual name was especially adored by the women with zero daughters. The mothers, including my own mother, made an agreement that the first woman to have a girl could name her daughter "Melody" and rest easy knowing no one else in their social circle would do the same.

As you've guessed, my parents were the first to have a girl.

When my maternal grandfather was told what my name was, he replied, "I hope she's not tone deaf." Unfortunately Grandpa Syd did not live long enough to know that music became a big part of my life. Arthur Sydney Simpson, my mom's dad, died when I was only three years old. The only memories I have of Grandpa Syd are things my mom told me about growing up in Transcona, a suburb of Winnipeg, and from family slideshows.

I know Grandpa Syd was a great gardener and grew not only vegetables but beautiful flowers too. Grandpa Syd's lush gardens were his music to the world. I am sure he would have been proud to know how much music shaped the notes of my life, especially when so many of my songs were eclipsed and shortened by illness and disease.

I did have the pleasure of knowing both my grandmothers. My father's mother lived well into her 70s despite being a widow for decades. (Dad's father died when my dad was only 16.) Mom's mom died just shy of 70. Memories of my grandmothers are brief. Those women were not exactly long lifers.

Forever Grateful

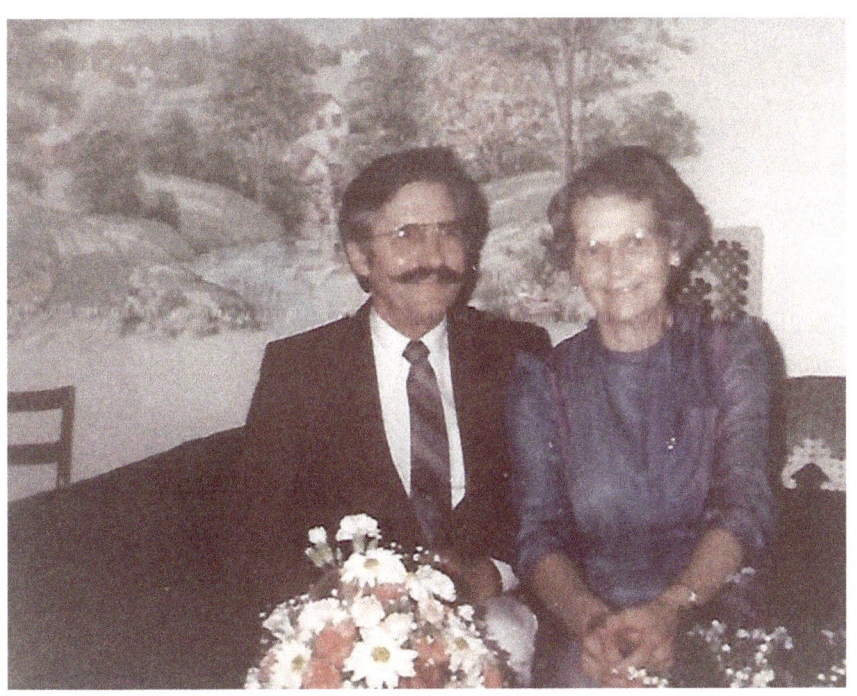

My mom and dad, date uncertain

Chapter 2

Music Is in the Marrow of My Bones

Music is love. Love is music. Music is life, and I love my life.
For as long as I can remember, music has played a beautiful role in my life. Vinyl records on our Hi-Fi. Singing in my church choir. Playing different instruments. I was always happiest when music was active in my life.

Our Hi-Fi was one of the central pieces of furniture in our living room. I believe each of us kids knew music as a force that was important and cherished in our household. We had no television, but we had our stereo. Music was either in the background or centre stage. From a very young age I considered music a friend, companion, and teacher.

Shortly after we moved to Peterborough, when I was three years old, I was diagnosed with mononucleosis. I ran a fever for six weeks straight. Our doctor came to the house regularly to check on me and reassured my parents that my health and vitality would bounce back. This was in the Dark Ages when doctors made house calls, knew their patients' names, and likely were a touch too positive about the impact of a long-term fever!

Looking back, I realize that a child with a high fever should have been taken to the ER within days, if not hours, of the thermometer hitting red. You don't need a medical degree to recognize that a full-blown and full-time fever is likely to damage a person's (especially a child's) internal organs. Today I realize that this fever signalled the beginning of my long-term poor health. A mysterious lack of energy and physical vitality would now accompany me throughout my life. It was only decades later when a specialist hypothesized that the initial damage to my kidneys occurred at three years old while I burned with fever at home.

When you're a child all you know is that you feel sick and you're incapable of doing what others are doing. For me, there was no playing tag, riding a bike or learning to swim. All the activities and games my brothers and the neighbourhood children did were beyond the realm of my physical health and endurance.

There's a reason why most people with ongoing illness grow up feeling like outsiders. Some of us feel like we don't fit in with our families. Oftentimes school is a disaster academically and socially because of our poor health and chronic absenteeism. Then there are those of us burdened with the curse of never aligning with who and what we are in the world.

Sickness banished me to the couch. Although throughout my childhood I was regularly propped up on pillows looking spoiled (my brothers' long-held view), I was actually being forced to look out passively and sadly at life. Even as a young child I knew there were activities, friendships, and joys closed to me because of my poor health.

But even in sickness there was music. Every morning my mom would carry me downstairs from my bedroom on the second floor and lay me on the couch so she could keep an eye on me. Mom didn't want me to feel alone or isolated. I would be dressed for the day, usually in a dress, since one of my mother's delights in life was celebrating the femininity of her one-and-only daughter. As we'd reach the bottom of the stairs, my stomach would heave. The smell of my parents' coffee always disagreed with me. Even today, decades later, I've never developed a taste for coffee!

Once my brothers were off to school, Mom would choose a record, and music would commence for the day. The music was always classical, religious, or light classics. It was comforting hearing Mom bustling around the kitchen or living room, humming and singing along to the record. During autumn while most kids returned to school or looked forward to Halloween, I looked out our bay window and admired the changing leaves. The days and weeks passed as I lay there, the leaves changing from green to red then gold.

In Peterborough there was a lovely baby grand piano in our living room. I have no idea where this beauty came from but any totem of music always made me feel at home. Six years later, as 1965 unfolded, the piano came with us when we moved again, this time to Alberta. I assume it was up to my mom to ensure that the movers were especially careful with the piano. Yet for whatever reason, this mysterious piano was left behind the following year when we moved to Toronto.

As you can see, moving around the country was just part of growing up inside a minister's family. Preachers rarely stayed at one church for more than five years. In fact, I believe it was protocol in some denominations that the minister and his family move every few years.

Too bad that as children we do not always appreciate what we have. For example, the baby grand that greeted me in Peterborough ultimately changed my life. Within a few years of our move from Moose Jaw to Peterborough, I began taking piano lessons. At seven years old, I clearly had no idea what a big deal it was to have one's very own baby grand piano! We'd had a piano in Moose Jaw too so a piano in our new home was nothing to get too excited or appreciative about. Music was like air to me; always around, plentiful, and life-affirming.

I would love to have a baby grand now. There is just something so regal about this majestic instrument. Of course, if you have the room and money in your life, I'd offer up one piece of advice: upgrade your baby grand and treat yourself to a full-size grand piano. There is something so magical and romantic about the piano irrespective of style or price tag. But a baby grand is absolutely a classic black beauty with class and panache.

Piano lessons were a requirement in our family. My parents could read music and both were excellent singers. My brothers were expected to take piano lessons until high school, at which point they were allowed to choose a different instrument to play in the school band. David chose the trumpet, Tim the trombone, and Jay the bassoon.

Despite the long-held tradition, by the time I reached high school neither Mom nor Dad expected me to quit piano and take up a new instrument. I suppose my parents recognized that I'd found a true love so why insist on changing the "keys" to my musical, piano-loving heart?

Sadly, I have no memory of how my first couple of piano lessons went. I do remember practising every day, which shows tremendous resolve considering I was only seven. Mom always made it so clear that she was happiest when my brothers and I practised our music without being reminded. Pleasing my mother by playing piano was a win/win for both her and me.

Week after week, lessons went along and I progressed in my knowledge and capabilities on the piano. Much as I enjoyed making music and learning the mysteries of written music, I was not comfortable performing. I was a shy, reserved child who loved to play but borderline hated the obligatory piano performances.

At the end of every year, my teacher hosted a recital. Students were expected to get dressed up and play in front of parents and friends. It seemed like everyone else was fine with playing their one or two musical pieces. When my turn came my hands would shake and my stomach would flip-flop. But I always seemed to make it through the performance, often overwhelmingly relieved I was no longer in the spotlight and on centre stage.

It was not until I was a lot older that playing in public became easier. Once I began speaking in public about organ donation and transplantation, a personal mission I was passionate about, I was finally able to overcome my performance fears. Advocating for others guided me to hit the right notes on stage as I learned to balance my confidence with my creativity.

Here is something I know for sure: my life today would be much less fulfilled if I did not have music. I know that now but when I was young, music was just part of our routine, which I recognized on some level as vital to our family and social circle. Music was a bridge (pun alert!), something special I shared with my parents and each of my brothers. And music was one of the few notes sweet enough and strong enough to connect me with the outside world.

Remember, I was often alone and isolated and unwell. My poor health sometimes made me feel that I had no special songs inside of me. Happily, I have come to know music is within me and around me. Music is in the marrow of my bones.

Chapter 3

School and Sick Notes

My school days were always filled with change and shifting social circles. As a family we moved regularly and religiously, which was fitting since Dad was a minister. His vocation was the reason for all our moves and school changes.

Womb life and cradle life happened in Moose Jaw. But school days, starting with kindergarten, kicked off in Peterborough. Grade 4 was endured in a little Alberta community called Wetaskiwin. The most surprising thing about Grade 4 was that, for the very first time, there was another "Melody" in my class. What are the chances of having two "Melody" girls in one class? My mother and her friends back in Moose Jaw would have been horrified! Mom had been assured her daughter would be the one and only Melody. To this day, I have never met another Melody and I admit I like being the only melody playing in the room.

The following year our family left the West for Toronto, where my parents purchased their first home. By the time I graduated Grade 5, I knew Grades 6 to 8 would be spent elsewhere. New neighbourhoods, new schools, new social circles. The shifting environments were often exhausting, but as fate would have it, I consider Grades 5 to 8 the happiest and best of my elementary years. It's no coincidence that my health during those years held strong and did not regularly banish me to the couch and away from my circle of friends.

I was a good student. I liked to learn, was eager to please, and have people like me. I was always ready to help a classmate with homework. Despite my being naturally shy and reserved, school was where I felt most comfortable and at ease. I made friends. I liked my teachers. I was included in activities. And I was continually grateful that I felt "normal" both physically and mentally.

Then it was time for high school. Most of my friends chose to attend the local school. My dad suggested that we check out the girls-only private schools. Why not? Apparently Dad had tried to convince my three brothers to attend a private high school but each son had declined. While Dad considered the private system better quality, more hands-on and possibly more shielded from the evils of the world, my brothers viewed their local public high school as more fun and less strict.

I knew Dad had been disappointed by the boys' decisions and I admit I didn't want to be another source of disappointment. Perhaps I was being altruistic when I told Dad I'd be happy and grateful to attend an all-girls school, where I knew no one and had zero concept of the social orbit I was crash-landing into: old money, tough cliques, strict curfews.

Since my dad was a minister, the majority of private schools offered a significant discount to clergy families. We never would have been able to afford my schooling without this discount, which reduced my tuition by approximately more than 50%. To put the tuition expense in context, today (2021) private schooling averages about $35 000 annually per student. If you're a student who boards at the school (i.e., lives in residence), your annual tuition tab weighs in at about $64 000 plus all fees, books, uniforms, etc.

Dad and I settled on Havergal (Anglican) College in Toronto, a short public transit commute from our new home, and where wealthy young women completed Grades 9 to 12. For the especially wealthy, little girls could attend Havergal as early as junior kindergarten, right up to Grade 8 and beyond. The school boasted about its exceptional programs ranging from the educational to the athletic to the extracurricular. Given that I was not much of a joiner, there were few clubs that appealed to me except for choir and piano, which I did join and enjoy.

Overall, I wish I could say attending Havergal had been wonderful. I would love to say I learned more there than I would have in the public school system. It would be lovely to gush about how the teachers were exceptional and kind, and provided me with a top-notch education and informed view of the world. But I do not feel that way at all.

I admit I considered Havergal a kind of "finishing school" where I was destined to get poshly educated, learn proper manners, and behave like a proper "young lady." Boy, was I wrong! So few of the young women were like me, and the differences extended well beyond social status.

Havergal exposed me to young women who swore like sailors. Most of them smoked all the time. They bragged about their promiscuity. And the top "queen bees," who were always from the richest and seemingly meanest families, regularly defied authority with contempt and callousness. Behaving in a mean or belligerent way toward teachers and/or peers was a game played for fun and popularity. To say I felt uncomfortable or horrified would be an understatement. My two years at Havergal, Grades 9 and 10, were an odd mixture of wishing I could fit in while simultaneously grateful I was nothing like the girls around me.

As for the education itself, I am sure it was adequate. I liked the majority of my teachers and most days I felt as if I was learning and growing. Fortunately, music continued to be part of my life while at Havergal. The school offered piano lessons, which I enrolled in immediately and attended regularly for the full two years I attended.

My first year at Havergal aligned with the school showcasing its first choir. Being accepted into the choir was an exciting moment for me. I was going to be a part of something! Acing the auditions was particularly sweet for me because my health continued to support rather than diminish me. I had the energy to practise before my audition and I had the stamina to show up to each and every choir rehearsal and recital. It was wonderful feeling so good and strong as I performed.

My first summer at Havergal the choir was offered the opportunity to go on tour for three weeks across Scotland and England. The choir mistress was from Great Britain and she'd arranged for us to sing in several famous cathedrals across the U.K. The cathedrals themselves were beautiful and majestic. The architecture, awe inspiring. Each day I was reminded of Canada's youthfulness when compared to countries with such hauntingly gorgeous places of worship. England's Coventry Cathedral in the West Midlands was my favourite. The cathedral had been bombed viciously throughout World War II and had never been fully repaired. Singing inside the cathedral's hallowed halls, I pretended the choir and I were serenading the soldiers who'd once worshipped there.

As I suspected, it didn't take long for me to feel homesick. Since I was a child I always felt more comfortable at home. I was never one for sleepovers. I'd tried to spend the night but usually my friend's mother would have to call my parents to come and take me home. Now that I was out of the country and touring, there were no phone calls home. No one was going to come and rescue me if I was feeling lonesome.

At every tour stop, there were letters waiting for me from Mom. She was so diligent and organized with her letter-writing and itinerary planning. The letters were always newsy: what the family was doing, how her job was going; anything she thought I might get a kick out of. I know Mom missed me as much as I missed her. Writing letters helped bridge the gap between us.

Once our choir finished our singing in Scotland and England, we spent a few days in Paris. It was amazing to be 16 and in Paris. Rather frightening but unforgettable. We stayed in a youth hostel, which was certainly eye opening for me. Living with other women in one large room with no real privacy anywhere, including the bathroom. I was surrounded by so many different types of people. Clearly, the girls and I were in an international and very cosmopolitan city. Every day I met people from all walks of life, from different countries far and wide. Being a sheltered white girl from a middle-class background, interacting with so many different cultures enriched and enthralled me. The world was so big!

Since our group was staying in Paris for only a couple of days, our choir mistress suggested we travel with only some of our belongings, leaving the majority of luggage at our London hotel. A friend and I shared a suitcase for our weekend in Paris. We were instructed to leave our luggage on the bus transporting us to Dover for the crossing to Calais, France. Yet once in France, my friend and I realized we had nothing. Our suitcase had vanished. We had no underwear, no toothbrush, no clean clothes. I greeted Paris with only the clothes on my back!

What pained me the most was that all the souvenirs I had purchased for my parents and brothers were gone too. The suitcase never reappeared despite the reassurances that it would. The other girls in the choir were generous in helping me and my friend out as best they could, but their clothes and hairbrushes were clearly not ours. Then and now, I was grateful to have received such generosity and kindness from the other choir members. Their help in Paris was certainly the nicest experience I had had with the majority of my Havergal peers.

Despite the luggage fiasco, I was still able to embrace the beauty and history of this amazing city: The Eiffel Tower, Notre Dame, L'Arc de Triomphe, the Louvre, and Versailles. Being with other girls of my age, who had much more life experience than I did, gave me deeper reserves of inner strength to explore new things. There was so much to see and do, and so little time.

Even when I was so young, sweet 16, I realized that time was always ticking. There were always two clocks running inside of me: the clock that measured my good days and the clock that measured the days and weeks, sometimes months, lost to illness and hospital stays.

(I returned to Paris when I was 54, travelling with a friend who'd grown up there. I must say, I enjoyed my time in 2010 even more than I had way back when I was 16 years old. Not only was I older and wiser, I had a better appreciation of what Paris was all about, especially the history and art.)

After that first year at Havergal, I was ready to return to the public high-school system but I didn't want to disappoint my dad or seem like a quitter. But the young women around me were so different from me that making meaningful connections was almost impossible. Most valued social connections, name brands, and their future (gorgeous) weddings. Nothing they chattered about appealed to me or inspired aspiration. We may have been in the same choir but my goodness, we were singing different songs about what life and love were about!

Happily, I did make one true friend while at Havergal. Her name was Marcia, and we lived in the same part of the city. We travelled back and forth together on public transit. We both "escaped" Havergal after completing Grade 10, and returned to the public education system. Sadly, I returned with a diagnosis that made the world stop spinning for me and my parents.

It was during my time at Havergal that I was first diagnosed with kidney disease. I began complaining about back pain shortly after turning 14. This was a new twist. The discomfort wasn't intense pain but there was certainly pressure on my back.

My doctor begrudgingly agreed to test my kidneys although she couldn't resist assuring my mother that kidney health had nothing to do with back pain. The doctor was proven wrong, which wasn't a win for anyone, especially me. Test results confirmed my kidneys were operating at less than 50%, which would surely account for my not feeling well. Toxins were steadily building up inside my system because my kidneys were unable to do what they do best: clean and protect.

At this point, I figured the medical people would be able to do something to make me feel better. Alas, this was not the case. I was not "sick enough." It was too soon for dialysis or any other form of targeted treatment. While some of my symptoms were treated with medication (e.g., despite barely being a teenager, I had high blood pressure), I was also told to change my diet. At 14, I was forced to stop eating anything salty, which, of course, included chips and popcorn!

Saddled with a new diagnosis and not physically feeling good at all, I returned to the public high-school system, Grade 11, to make another unfortunate discovery: the friends I had had in elementary school had found other friends. My one friend, Marcia, from Havergal attended the same high school, but we didn't have a single class together. Despite our getting together on weekends, I was once again back to feeling as if I were living life from inside a bubble. I was sick and I was excluded from so much because of my poor health. There were days when it was hard not to fall prey to self-pity and self-loathing. As I look back, I feel even more compassion for the 14-year-old girl I once was. I had health problems, social problems, and was also burdened with changing hormones too! Despite everything, I continued to be a good student and managed to graduate high school with a B+ average.

Music continued to guide me.

Rather than going to college or university, I chose to study piano full-time. I found a wonderful teacher, George McElroy, a lovely middle-aged man who had devoted his life to music and teaching. I was 18, studying piano, and living at home. My health, if I had to rate it out of 10, ranged between a miserable four to an okay-so-far seven, depending on the day.

George was a soft-spoken man, who knew his music inside out. He was caring but ready to push me along in my studies. He expected things from me that I was not sure I would be able to accomplish, which was always an indication I was learning and growing. When I went outside my comfort zone and took a risk on a piece, George and I were proud. His teachings and mentorship made me more of a risk taker not just on the keys of our piano but in life as well.

George believed in me. Not that other people in my life didn't, but I knew I could talk to George about my music dreams and challenges, and trust that he'd give me an honest, positive answer.

One of my favourite composers was, and still is, Claude Debussy. As I studied with George, I chose to perform Debussy pieces whenever possible. My least favourite composer to play, then and now, is J.S. Bach. I respect his compositions and his talent, but his creations are so ridiculously hard to play!

As fate would have it, I was obligated to play Bach every time I advanced a piano grade (I studied until Grade 10) so my foe eventually became a friend. Playing a Bach piece always signified that George and I had hit another milestone: I had advanced in my piano studies and increased my confidence on stage and as a performer.

As I write about George, I smile. As his young student, I always called him "Mr. McElroy." We ran into one another a few years ago while I was attending a concert with my daughter, Lauren. I introduced my lovely piano teacher as "Mr. McElroy" despite him insisting he be called "George." I couldn't bring myself to do it, wanting to show my teacher and mentor as much respect and reverence as I could.

Always gracious and encouraging, George expressed real delight when I told him Lauren was following in my musical footsteps. I resisted telling him that I believe Lauren is "Mr. McElroy" to many of her students too;

encouraging growth and risk taking while inviting students to express themselves authentically and powerfully through music.

Working with George as I prepared for the Royal Conservatory of Music exams gave my life a direction and structure that it would not have had otherwise. There were not many other parameters in my life, no job, no relationship. Without piano practising, my days would have been long and tedious, especially since there were so many days (weeks, really) when physically I felt unwell.

Every day was a blessing when there was time for practising, for studying music theory, for crocheting or knitting. Going on an outing was always sweet, especially if I was able to have lunch with Mom while she was at work or venturing out for a walk with her, depending on my energy level.

I used to carry around the assumption that I had somehow settled or compromised when I chose to study piano and not go to college or university. I think differently now. Music had always called to me and I chose to follow that call, which enriched me as a person. Dedicating myself to music made me kinder, braver, and stronger. I wish the same style of life path for my children and grandchildren.

By deciding to study piano, I started on a musical path that continues today. It always amazes me how life works out.

Chapter 4

Keys to Creativity and Confidence

Summer 1978. I am 22 years old. Living with my parents while studying piano full time. Playing piano usually demanded more energy than I had, and those were tough, frustrating days.

Despite the "off" days with my health, making piano the professional focus of my life gave me the courage to start teaching students of my own. If I had concerns about my students, I'd confide in my teacher and mentor, Mr. McElroy. I felt grateful that my life's path was revealing itself one note, one student, one lesson at a time.

I advertised in the local paper and soon had a roster of a dozen players ranging in age from six to 40-ish. Since I lived at home with few overhead expenses, teaching was a flexible and easily profitable enterprise. I kept my student numbers low so that I would have enough energy for my own musical studies, which ranged from piano practising to exam preparation. Teaching gave my life structure, purpose, and moments of deep joy.

By the time Christmas rolled around, I'd been teaching students for about four months. I could tell I was feeling good mentally and emotionally because I decided that year to make all my Christmas presents by hand. Thanks to my thriving teaching business and my private study with Mr. McElroy, both my confidence and creativity were sky-high.

As usual there were weekly and sometimes daily physical setbacks, but my mindset was strong and positive. The Christmas gifts I made that year were either knitted, crocheted, or sewn. Crafting gifts for those I loved was a positive use of my time and energy. There was satisfaction in knowing I had accomplished something no matter how I felt physically. No matter how lonesome or lost I might feel.

Not only did having students give structure to my days, my teaching business gave me consistent social interaction. I always looked forward to seeing my students. One of my students, Stephen, was seven years old and so cute and engaging. After he had been taking lessons for a few weeks, Stephen's dad decided he wanted to learn how to play piano too. What a pleasure having a father-son duo as students. My teaching developed and deepened exponentially because it was so challenging to find teachable moments (and songs!) that engaged a boy under 10 and a man under 50!

There were students who, of course, had no interest in music, piano, or practising. There was one little girl who came and stared longingly out the window at the park behind my parents' house. She definitely did not want to be inside with me and my piano lessons. After weeks of lacklustre lessons for us both, I finally plucked up the courage to tell her parents they needed to save their money and find something their daughter actually loved and enjoyed doing.

Once you become a teacher, whether standing at the front of a traditional classroom or sitting down beside a student on a piano bench, you realize just how much time, energy, and effort teaching demands. But (deep) learning demands just as much energy as (good) teaching does.

I was delighted to discover that the few adult students I taught were some of my "best" students because they were happy to learn, enthusiastic to practise, and grateful for guidance and encouragement. The adults were both humble and patient as they learned. Adult students sat beside me on that piano bench because they wanted to be there, not because someone they loved told them they better sit there, practise, and learn!

I always felt such tremendous compassion for the kids forced to take lessons with me. What the kids never realized was that the half hour-long lessons felt excruciatingly slow for me too. No one was having fun, not the kid and not me. The young students who loved to play? Those lessons sped by and I always felt a bit lost after the lesson was over. If the student moved on to a more advanced teacher, I was sad to see them go and grow elsewhere. But the show must go on, right?

Teaching or not, young or old, married or single, happy or sad, there has always been music in my life. I played piano to my children when they were still in utero. I sang to them once they were born. And we sang together as mother-and-baby and later as mother-and-grown child. I wouldn't change a single second of those singing-and-playing memories with my kids.

When my son Shamus was about three years old, he tapped me on the hand as I was playing the piano. He asked me to play "that" piece. "Which piece?" I asked him. "You know the one, Mommy." Shamus stood close to the piano bench. I patted his curly blond hair and gazed into his big brown eyes. Shamus looked very seriously and intently at me, expectant. I wasn't sure which tune he wanted, but I started playing a Mozart sonata, a favourite to play when I was pregnant with him. Shamus' face broke into a big smile followed by a giggle. Imagine. The boy had heard this song, and savoured its impact, before he was even officially here on Earth with us. Amazing.

When Lauren was still en route to Earth, I'd sing "All Through the Night," a song Emma, Lauren's niece (my granddaughter), asks me to sing today whenever the grand-girlies sleep over at our place. The tradition of singing and listening is being passed on and I couldn't be happier that our family song continues across the generations.

Just like a family tree, music branches out and grows stronger in my life as I grow older. Relationships, houses, hobbies. Things come and go, but music always remains. I suppose my name was a signifier early on that I'd be a lover of music.

Several years ago a dear friend of mine started calling me "Melodious," my first-ever nickname that to this day makes me smile and almost blush. (My hit-and-miss school career could have inspired the nickname "Absent" since I so rarely attended school because of my health!) As I grew up and older, I discovered another new love that was both melodious and magnificent. I adored a brand-new, passionate love... and still remained happily married!

In the fall of 1988 Lauren was still a baby and Shamus was six years old. Bob, Lauren's dad, had a work conference in Connecticut and I was able to go with him, a treat for us both. My mom looked after the kids while Bob and I enjoyed a weekend away. At one of the posh corporate dinners, I met a young woman playing a full-sized (grand) harp. I was immediately enchanted by the instrument. I had never seen a harp up close. When the talented musician took a break from playing, I introduced myself by complimenting her beautiful playing. After chatting for about 15 minutes, she offered to be my teacher. I love Americans, they know how to hustle. Remember this was the late 80s, long before video conferencing, FaceTime or Facebook. There was no way she could teach me from Connecticut while I lived in Toronto! Both of us were disappointed but where there's a will, there's a way.

The blessing of that entire trip, and that kind and gracious woman, was that she invited me into the possibility that I could, somehow, with courage and creativity, learn to play the harp. Being a stay-at-home mom was a dream and a delight, but I needed a musical outlet, something new and exciting to learn that would challenge me and relieve stress too.

Which instrument to take up at the ripe ole age of 33? And that would help me kick off another New Year? The harp, of course. Next big question? Where does one get a harp? And once you have one, where do you find a patient and kind harp teacher? After a few phone calls and chats with friends, success. I leased a harp for three months and hired a harp teacher willing to teach me once a week at her home. After my three-month trial with the harp, I committed to two things enthusiastically: I'd buy the harp and I'd study with my teacher for one year. I was back to being a student and found tremendous stress relief by living inside a "beginner's mind" once a week for an hour. When I was playing the harp, I was not a full-time mother but a full-time musician. I believe those lessons, that creative respite, made me a better mom, daughter, and wife.

Because I had played piano for so many years, playing the harp came fairly easily since both piano and harp use treble and bass clefs. I chose to play a Celtic harp as opposed to a Grand harp because the Celtic harp is significantly smaller. (As you likely know, I am not a large or physically strong person!) Another reason the Celtic harp called to me was cost.

Depending on the make and the number of strings, a Celtic harp costs somewhere between $1,000 and $6,000. An investment, indeed. But a Grand harp starts around $10,000 and just keeps going up in price. If you get to the place where you are going to take harping seriously and need a top-of-the-line harp, you can pay as much as $180,000. Too much for my budget.

That first harp teacher was an excellent harpist and playing was her life's calling. She was a professional harpist who played mostly on the Grand harp. I believe that playing the harp was what gave her life meaning. One could not help but respect her passion and purpose. I, on the other hand, was studying and playing only as a stress-relieving, happiness-inducing hobby. I had children who needed looking after and my time to practise was limited. My teacher took playing and teaching seriously. A touch too seriously. There were weeks when I had had little time to practise and had not made much progress with the pieces I was working on. Suzanna had little patience for what she considered my "feeble excuses."

These "excuses" included looking after my children, my husband, as well as taking good care of myself so I wouldn't end up in hospital. Despite bouts of mild irritation at her lack of empathy, I understood my teacher's views. Our lives and priorities were very different. My harp teacher was a healthy woman. I was not blessed with good health most days, so my life followed that diseased trajectory. I had good days and I had bad days. I thought it was a compliment to both my harp and my teacher that when I was having a good, healthy day, I chose to practise!

As fate would have it, after a year studying with her and sharing too many of my "feeble excuses," I concluded I needed a new teacher and mentor. I wanted someone who could come to my house and who realized (and respected) that I was playing harp as a hobby and creative outlet. I was not interested in being a professional musician, but I was looking for self-development and joy.

Believe it or not, there is such a thing as a harp community, which quickly put me in touch with a teacher willing to make house-harp calls. What a difference to stay in my own home, close to my kids, and play music. I always looked forward to lessons with Sharlene, who patiently and kindly deepened my love for the sound and feel of the harp. Young Lauren and Shamus were enthusiastic and well-behaved (for the most part) cheerleaders and musical judges during my lessons. Funny to imagine that Sharlene and I started working together over 30 years ago.

My children are now all grown up, yet they still sit and cheerlead whenever they catch me playing the harp. I am grateful Sharlene and I have remained friends. You would think that over the years I would have perfected changing harp strings by myself, but not so. I still periodically send out an S.O.S. to Sharlene to come and rescue me, and she never lets me down. I am so fortunate to have such a lovely and generous friend, and I am grateful my long-time teacher has become a long-time friend.

Ironically, my original stance that harp playing was a hobby, not a profession has shifted. My love and enjoyment of the harp inspired me to transition into professional harp playing, which means I play (and get paid) professionally. Right from the beginning I didn't know how to charge for gigs. Since I had no intention of making my living by being a harper, I was uncertain of my worth. I tried to make it so that the client could give me some idea of their budget. To this day I still have difficulty deciding what to charge, but happily my heart and the client's budget always find common ground.

Over the years I've played at wedding ceremonies, event receptions, house parties, and a number of funerals. One of my favourite playing experiences was harping at the annual Garden Tour in Toronto's East End, the famous Beach neighbourhood. Musicians, whether playing alone like me or with others, are asked to play in a magnificent private garden while guests savour the gorgeous flowers and foliage.

For several years Garden Tour organizers asked me to play my harp in the refreshment area. My listeners were always happy and appreciative. Like me, they appreciated beauty and blooms, fine wine and cheese. My audience was always respectful and complimentary. A kind audience is immunity against stage fright and worst-case scenario thinking.

The worst experience I recall is playing at a reception in a fancy hall. There were people all around and someone came and stood right in front of my harp with their back to me. Let's just say that the person was as large as I am small! I was completely overshadowed by this nasty "patron of the arts"! Not once did they turn around or acknowledge I was playing. I certainly do not expect people to "ooh" and "aah" over the music or the musician (merry me) but I am a human being and as such deserve to at least be acknowledged. Plus, being gracious to the musicians at an event is just good manners. Ask my kids: they've been trained in the fine art of giving and receiving musical praise.

One reason this nasty experience sticks out in my mind, and still bothers me just a bit, is when I was playing and being ignored by that person (likely in a totally unmalicious but clueless way), I was reminded of all the times I was sick and unable to participate in activities, events, or gatherings. When you are sickly, you are often ignored and the invisibility is a stab to the soul.

Perhaps this is why I have such a hard time being overlooked or ignored in public places. I am not a big person physically and I realize it is possible that I am easy to miss. But when people walk right past me, or actually bump into me without acknowledging me, I do get upset. I have come to realize that most people are just unaware when they ignore or overlook others. We're all so busy inside our minds that people and places are encountered with careless cruelty at times. Funny the wounds we carry.

My over-sensitivity to "big people" stomping on my "little person" is absolutely rooted in those decades of being sick and feeling excluded. When you're unable to participate in life events, especially the joyful ones, you really do feel like you are insignificant and a nothing. I'm grateful every time I make someone "invisible" feel seen, heard, and understood. And when I see my kids show compassion and patience to others easily overlooked? Words can't express my relief and gratitude for helping raise such kindly humans. We all want to belong. So, it's our job to extend a helping hand and open a closed heart. As I write that, I realize I sound like a sensitive, overly emotional artist! A musician looking for mischief, which makes me smile. Music has always been the bridge between self-expression and the whole gamut of my emotions whether my greatest joys or deepest sorrows.

Music gifted me with one of the most poignant times of my life back in 2000, a year I will never forget. My father was dying. Since there was no viable cancer treatment left to offer him in hospital, Dad asked to go home to die.

My dad was then remarried to a lovely woman named Pat, who was loving, kind, and generous as well as madly in love with my dad. I had the privilege of bringing my harp into their home and playing for my dad as he passed from this world to the next. What a gift to help my dad transition. To bear witness to him leaving both his body and his loved ones behind. I will always treasure Pat for making the decision to bring Dad home and for allowing me to sit with him for hours. My music offered Dad some peace while he lay in his bed and began the hard work of saying goodbye and letting go.

Dad and I certainly had our differences over the years, but we'd grown close. For example, Dad took great delight in pointing out to me, as I played harp for him, that the flowers in his room were from my brother Jay's garden, gorgeous irises and peonies. He confided that he wanted to be cremated and his ashes spread in Jay's garden. Dad would look at the flowers, smile and say, "That's where I am going to be, enjoying the flowers." My dad had nurtured and tended to beautiful roses in his front- and backyards for years.

I'm grateful I could focus on playing as Dad shared his final sentiments with me. I'm afraid if I hadn't been playing, I might have hysterically cried and wailed. But perhaps not. My father looked to the afterlife with a mix of fascination and agitation. The flowers I sat beside as well as his decision to have the garden be his final resting place soothed him and made him happy as he reflected on his life, his decisions, and his relationships.

Safe passage, Dad.

My mom had remarried and was living in Manitoba around the time my dad died. Mom was always so happy to have me play when I went to visit her. I made a point of playing every day we were together. Even on the days I didn't really feel like it, I played for her and sang to her too. What you do for love, especially a mother's love. Playing music became even more important to Mom's emotional wellness after her stroke. Both of us mourned not living in the same city and being so far away from one another.

The stroke limited Mom's ability to really get out much so it was a special treat for her to hear me play. I'd always pack a book of hymns in my luggage and sometimes she would sing along as I played my harp. Obviously, my mother knew the majority of my songs and my repertoire since she was the woman who immersed me in music from an early age. Whenever Mom would recognize a tune, a smile would break open on her beautiful face. One of her very favourite pieces was "The Spinning Wheel," a folksy song made popular by John McDermott. Even to this day when I play it, privately or professionally, I always preface the song by saying out loud, "This is for you, Mom."

At one time I had a total of three harps: a small one I'd take to Manitoba so I could play for Mom; one I had bought from a harp maker in Oakville; and my pride and joy created by a harp maker in Winnipeg. The first time I heard one of Larry Fisher's harps, I knew I wanted one. Immediately. Larry built harps in his basement workshop in Winnipeg. Fortunately for me, his workshop was near the airport, which I frequented somewhat regularly on my way to see Mom. Larry was generous and gracious with his time. I learned a lot about harp making, especially as he crafted more than one harp at a time. I could watch the different stages and processes of his mastery.

I've been asked more than once why I didn't teach my kids how to play the harp or piano. In simplest terms, my kids can be fairly stubborn. Even though I had my Grade 10 RCM (Royal Conservatory of Music) in piano, according to my teenage kids, I didn't really know anything. Life at our home was just better and more peaceful if I didn't mandate piano lessons. Instead, Lauren and Shamus took piano lessons elsewhere and I didn't mind a bit. I prefer life to be as melodious as possible.

On that note, it's a real shame when I see so many of my peers without music in their lives or when I see music study slashed from education budgets. Music is such a deep source of joy. For me, music has been a type of medicine too. Not only do I enjoy playing piano and harp, I adore singing in church and community choirs. When you are part of a church choir, you need to be always aware of what is coming next and making sure you have the right music. As much as I love singing, I am much more comfortable being in the congregation and singing out of the hymnal;

that way I can choose to sing harmony or not. One must not just sing the music but have the space to feel it too.

Lauren shares my passion. Years ago we joined a community choir for a fall session. Rehearsal nights were a great way to spend an evening together. Both of us loved being part of a group of singers supportive of each other, gathered to make music and have fun. Our musical director was a creative person with high expectations so our first concert was not simply a concert where we stood in rows, singing and wearing black pants and white tops. Instead, Lauren and I had the honour and privilege of being part of a production, complete with costumes, emotion, and movement. What fun and excitement! For me, music has always been therapeutic. Not only is music uplifting, the sound of music is good company when I am alone. Music has healed me many times and shown me how to express deep love, joy, and sorrow. Music has also helped me let go and live.

Chapter 5

From the Mountains to the Valley

In life, dreams come and go. As I was growing up, two dreams remained constant for me. One dream was that one day I would be a mother. The other, that I would have a husband and a home. The white picket fence, 2.5 children, something from the world of television and what most perceive as an attainable and sure-fire future.

When I was diagnosed with kidney disease at 17, I was told that I would never have children. One of the potential outcomes of kidney disease is difficulty getting pregnant or carrying a baby to term. When a body is struggling with kidney disease, it's working so hard managing hormone levels and general malaise that growing a fetus, nurturing a little one, is beyond the body's capacity. I remember feeling devastated when this news was delivered with authority and permanence by a well-meaning doctor. At a young age, I learned that life can swing sideways quickly and unapologetically.

In a moment, my motherhood dream was shattered. Life feels unfair and uninspiring when you associate motherhood going hand-in-hand with marriage and a man. I couldn't have babies so how was I ever going to attract and marry a man? (Times were different back then, remember.) Two beautiful dreams gone before I was 20 years old. Or so I was told.

As a teenager I had a few boyfriends. Shortly after my no-motherhood news, I started dating Drew. I was 18 years old and Drew a year younger. The scandal of dating a younger man! Drew and I met while we were in high school. We dated for a couple of years after graduation and then decided we'd get married. Because we were so young and inexperienced, we had never talked about having children, meaning that Drew was not aware that I might not be able to carry a child to term. Being engaged, life was unfolding in a way that seemed to promise I was to fulfill at least one dream: getting married and being a wife.

Committing to Drew felt like my one and only opportunity to get married. Maybe no one else would want me since I was constantly sick, weak, or dealing with acute health issues. I definitely felt like damaged goods. As I write those words, I grieve for that young woman and her low feelings of self-worth. I was looking for a place in the sun, a place or person that encouraged me to thrive not just survive. Just like now, as a young woman I drew tremendous strength and resolve from my religious faith and the belief that the universe is benevolent and affirmative.

I was raised on going to church, listening to gospel and classical music, playing piano, and reading lots of books. Drew's family did not go to church, had no real interest in music other than what was playing at the Legion on Saturday nights. Reading was considered a chore no longer valid since no one attended school anymore. If you had to define me in two words back then, I'd say "lifelong learner." Drew in two words? "Man's man." Opposites attract, indeed.

In my parents' home growing up and right into adulthood, none of us drank alcohol because of our religious beliefs as well as our modest social conventions. Drinking was one of the absolute no-nos according to our church, along with card playing, dancing, and rock-and-roll music. My fiancé, on the other hand, was raised in an environment where having a beer (or 12) was a mandatory family prerequisite at all social functions. Drew and his family were not bad people. Far from it. But they were not my kind of people and all of us knew there was a black sheep (me) not fitting in with the in-law herd.

As in life, our differences finally caught up to us, to me anyway. I knew I could not live my life being untrue to the person I was and dreamt of becoming. I wanted to attend church, listen to music, study piano, read books, and transform continually. My escape or expansion was not rooted in alcohol or dances but through my spirituality and connection to Source. I always felt most connected to spirit when I was sitting in the church pew and on the piano bench. I am, in essence, a solitary creature. There's a reason why reading was, and remains, one of my most passionate loves. Learning and growing were the ways I wanted to travel through the world, no matter how young or old (or sick!) I was.

My lifestyle choices were unfathomable to Drew and his family. I felt like I would have to give up too much to remain in our relationship so, months after getting engaged, I made a heart-breaking decision: I ended our engagement. I was grateful that Drew accepted the news with reverence and respect. Perhaps he too knew that our stars were not aligned. Relief is a powerful and welcome emotion when saying "no" so you can remain authentic and aligned with your destiny.

Of course, my timing could have been better. I broke up with Drew on New Year's Eve, the last night of 1977. My timing has never really been that good, except on the piano of course, but in the big picture? My really big choices have always been the right ones at the right time, and I'm grateful.

My parents had always been supportive of me and my life decisions. They were no different regarding my breakup with Drew. I never had the feeling they were unsupportive of my engagement, yet they were not disappointed when I unhitched from Drew and the life that awaited me.

As in any breakup, my heart took time to heal. Things were different. There was no one to go out with, no one to chat with every day. Life was lonely, which is especially terrible when you're a young woman of 21 living at home and rebounding, not just from heartache but chronic illness too.

To overcome the initial pain from the heartbreak, I went to my brother Jay's place in Hamilton. He and his wife were so accommodating and kind. A few days away from "the scene of the heart/hard crime" helped me grow stronger and less sad. Drew continued to call me and eventually I tried my best to explain why I chose to leave and move forward without him.

My father likely sensed I was feeling as if I were damaged goods, a state of mind not foreign to me. I moped around the house for weeks after the breakup, diligently doing the heavy lifting of healing and grieving. But nothing stays the same, does it? The good or the bad. Sunshine did return to my life, and I was grateful for its warmth.

In 1979, approximately two years after the breakup, Dad and I took a summer cross-country road trip. As we travelled from Toronto to Vancouver, I felt good, inside and out. Dad was in high spirits during the drive and had eased nicely into the 55th year of his life. His co-pilot (me) was 23 and finally feeling good about the future. Being from a family of boys, having my dad to myself for more than three weeks was a treat and a delight.

We took turns driving the family car, a giant burgundy Buick Lebaron. We stopped off in Lake Louise to see my best friend Marcia, who was working as a manager at the Lake Louise Inn. While Dad continued on to Vancouver, Marcia and I remained in Alberta. We had a wonderful time together and my love of the mountains was rekindled immediately. (Remember, we used to live in Alberta.) I was in pretty good shape on the health front, able to enjoy each day with no ill effects. I felt strong, young, and free. Not only did I enjoy my time with Marcia, I met several eligible men. What a thrill to once again flirt, feel pretty, and have men interested in me.

After spending a week with Marcia, I took the train to Vancouver to meet up with my father. Dad had settled into Vancouver life while taking some university courses as part of his personal and spiritual growth. Like father, like daughter. Both of us were passionate lifelong learners.

I arrived in the big city with a secret I was eager to share with Dad.

On that train trip through the mountains, on the rails between Calgary and Vancouver, I made the momentous decision to leave my parents' home, move out West, and live life on my own terms, whether in sickness or in health. It was time for me to spread my wings and really fly away from the nest, something I had never felt inclined to do before.

My time in Lake Louise had inspired me to realize that there was more to life than living at home, playing it safe, and dreaming small. It was time to take a risk and approach life as an amazing adventure, not a sickly sentence. This new worldview was such a change from what I had believed would be my life path. Yes, a part of me was scared to death, but the other half cheered and roared with excitement! I also knew that if I didn't take this chance to head West and live in Calgary, I never would. It was now or never.

As I travelled on the train toward the West Coast and my dad, I knew I was at a crossroads about who I was going to be in this lifetime. I chose a new life direction from a place of strength and faith. Plus, I knew myself well. If I chose to only move out of my childhood home and get my own place in Toronto, the option of moving back with Mom and Dad would be so easy. By living in far-away Calgary, I would not easily be able to go back to my old life.

I was choosing to "burn the ships" and commit. Go big or go home. I wasn't big but I wasn't going home again. The time had come to truly live and feel alive. I knew I had no job, no place to live, and no money. But I did have resources and, more importantly, I was resourceful.

Opportunities arose as I stepped into my dream. There were relatives and family friends in Calgary, who immediately and graciously offered to host me as I looked for a job, home, and life. Marcia cheered me on from Lake Louise, my best friend only 90 minutes away from my to-be home in Calgary! Our hobby of meeting men and getting into (wholesome) mischief could continue unabated.

Within weeks of returning to Toronto with Dad, I packed up my little red Honda Civic. I pointed my life compass West, just like I had decided, just like I had promised myself. What an adventure. Looking back, I am amazed by that young woman's courage, craziness, and grit. All my earthly belongings went with me: stereo, dishes, clothes, my Bentwood rocker.

There were tears shed by Mom and by me. We held each other tight. Being the amazing woman she was, Mom never stood in my way, despite how difficult and scary it must have been for her, seeing her only girl, with less than stellar health, moving so far away. She knew I had no intention of ever returning full-time to my childhood home. The sickly bird had flown the nest via a tiny red car and the epic TransCanada Highway.

I have a number of memories of that solo cross-country trip. For those of you who've driven from Ontario out West, you well know that Ontario is one very large province. I couldn't believe how long it took me to escape my home province! I spent one night at a cheap motel. The next night with a great uncle in northern Ontario, in Thunder Bay. The next day,

I finally made my way into rural Manitoba where I stayed with my aunt (my mother's sister) and her husband. (As a side note about how strange life can be: years after my visit, my aunt died, making her husband a widower. My widowed uncle eventually asked my divorced mother to marry him! Two sisters married to the same man, but not at the same time! True story.)

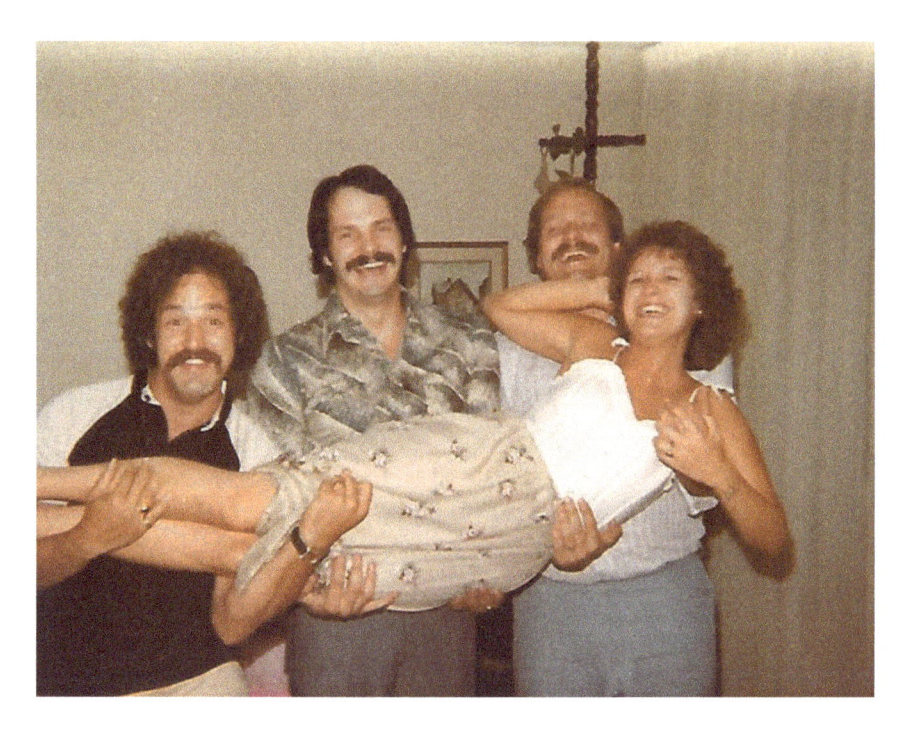

Me and my brothers just before I left for Calgary, 1979
(L to R) Tim, Jay, David, Me

In Calgary, I settled in with my dad's side of the family, a lovely aunt and uncle. Within weeks of my arrival I was living downtown, housesitting for a friend. Despite having a beautiful home to stay in (for free), job hunting proved challenging. The only work experience I had was working in a grocery store, working on a switchboard, and teaching piano. What was nice? The same week I found an apartment, I found a job. Yamaha Music was looking for a piano teacher. I snipped out the newspaper ad, took a deep breath, and called the phone number. I had to work hard to convince the woman on the other end of the phone that my name truly was, pinky swear promise, "Melody."

Working at Yamaha was a whole different experience from teaching at home. There was a prescribed curriculum, and I was expected to work with a class rather than one-on-one with students. There were times when I felt I was in way over my head because I was unfamiliar with the Yamaha curriculum, as well as its corporate culture.

I certainly knew more piano than any of my students and I could easily play difficult pieces upon request. But Yamaha's philosophy of teaching really challenged me. I had to balance their corporate teaching principles with my creative teaching beliefs. The company and the new teacher had extremely different teaching styles. For example, Yamaha expected its teachers to mentor music students through timely instruction, comprehensive musical training, group lessons (only), and exclusive use of Yamaha materials. Contrast those rigid guidelines with my experience teaching students one-on-one at home. Back in Toronto I worked independently and crafted lessons as I went along. I was committed to matching my students' lessons with their personality, learning style, and creative goals. Adapting to the Yamaha curriculum often humbled me because of the steep learning curve. But overall that awkwardness made me a better and more patient teacher, and a more confident performer too. I was learning right alongside my students!

I had the basics for setting up house in Calgary. I was able to get a bed, a small table, and one chair from a friend. Complete homeyness. I was comfortable and content in my own space while also enjoying the company of new friends. I befriended a colleague, a New Zealander, and we'd regularly spend Saturday nights in my apartment, sitting on the floor, drinking wine (me?) while listening to music and wondering where all the eligible guys were. (We agreed they were sitting at home, drinking beer, and wondering where all the eligible girls were!) Alcohol was still new to me when I lived in Calgary but like so many young people, I thought drinking wine with girlfriends (or on a date) was a sign of independence and a way to break away from family influence.

Life was good. I was happy. I felt sophisticated and was having fun. I had a life. My health was as good as it could be. I was making the most of my physical vitality and strength. There was something about Calgary that felt special and fit me perfectly. Calgary was still very much "Cow Town" in 1979 and possessed a rugged Western energy that kept the city, and me, going. I made the most of having my own place, living my own life, making my own decisions. I was making a go of this new endeavour and felt proud of myself. My parents and brothers cheered me on from Toronto, so I felt free but still rooted and loved too.

My health still demanded attention and maintenance. I met regularly with a nephrologist in Calgary, a kidney specialist, and it was he who first introduced me to the term "kidney transplant." I was assured that I'd need a new kidney within a few years, long before I turned 30. I knew nothing about organ transplantation at the time. My immediate reaction was that there was no way anyone was going to cut me open! I was definitely afraid of surgery, especially since I had so rarely gone "under the knife." I had been spared that type of pain and suffering, at least until now.

I knew I was in trouble soon after visiting my family for Christmas. Once I was back in Calgary and just weeks into 1980, I could tell that my health was gearing up to fail me once again.

All through January I did the best I could to keep up with life. I went to work. I grocery shopped. I went to bed early and rose late. Every day I was more and more depleted in energy, physically and emotionally. What was happening? Why was it happening? I was not ready to admit defeat and go to the hospital or call my mom. But reality became undeniable. My health was deteriorating. By mid-February, I could no longer drag myself to work. I knew I had hit a new threshold, a new rock bottom, regarding my kidney function. The organ had never performed this poorly or behaved this badly. I was literally and figuratively going toxic.

One of the reasons for fatigue in kidney disease is anemia, a shortage of oxygen carrying red blood cells. The damaged kidneys can no longer produce a hormone called erythropoietin (EPO), which tells the bone marrow to produce new red blood cells. Without new cells, my body had less oxygen, so I was increasingly tired, cold, and unable to focus. Toxins were building in my body, and my body was giving me just about every signal it could that my ship was heading into the rocks.

Even though I knew what to expect when I got "sick," it did not make my anger and frustration any less real. I had been doing so well. I had been taking good care of myself. I was able to keep up with my job, sleeping well, and eating healthy. I had taken such a huge risk moving out West. My risk-taking had paid off and gifted me a life on my terms: a good, fun, meaningful life. And now I was about to fall flat on my face because of something I couldn't control or even see, my substandard kidneys. I felt such rage and shame. Self-pity and sadness.

I called my family to tell them I might need a kidney transplant. My brother Tim immediately volunteered to be tested. He knew nothing about the donor process except that he wanted to help his little sister. Tim and I had always been close. On one level, I deeply appreciated his love and kindness yet the joy (and relief) was overshadowed. My Calgary world was shrinking fast. I could feel independence slipping from me. My reaction to Tim's "gift of life" offer was muted by the grief of having to go home. There's hopelessness inside the assessment that you've failed or, worse, concluding that you're a failure.

Only years later did I learn that my oldest brother, David, had also wanted to be my donor but his poor heart health precluded him from even being tested as a potential match. There was so much love, selflessness, and care extended to me during this time, but I was blind to most of it. Pain does that, casting shadows over our sources of light and joy. In retrospect, I realize now that my kidney dysfunction was showing me, once again, how to live and what, and whom, to stay mindful of when life ships lemons all over you.

Despite my being actively sick for the majority of my life, my family could not fully understand how kidney disease limited my life. My family considered my returning home as a positive "fix" or solution to a problem. But kidney disease was a robber and a thief. The disease stole so much from me in so many ways from the mundane (e.g., never having the energy or strength to be athletic) to the major (e.g., an inability to live independently and without surgery). Perhaps the disease's biggest theft was my self-confidence and self-worth. Seeing yourself as "damaged goods" and likely "unlovable goods" is neither healthy nor empowering. I am grateful I eventually outgrew such terrible labels, but I know feeling damaged has cost me. Illness has forever altered how I view myself and others.

What does it mean for someone like me to "get sick"? When most people get sick, they think of the flu or a cold. When I get acutely sick, usually an escalation or deepening of my general health malaise, I feel lethargic and nauseated. My skin becomes itchy. I sleep too much or not enough. Getting out of bed and facing the day are difficult undertakings.

During those last few weeks in Calgary, there were days when all I could do was move from the bed to my rocking chair and back again. My thinking was slow and foggy. Those kidneys that had served me so well, for the most part, were shutting down and making me sick. I was no longer able to teach piano so bye-bye to earning money and enjoying financial independence. I couldn't pay my rent. Once I knew I was unable to work and earn money, it was only a matter of time until I returned home. My kidneys had defeated me.

I tearfully gave notice at the music studio. I wasn't the only person who cried, so that was nice. Afterwards, I returned to my apartment and waited for my dad to bring me back home. Dad flew to Calgary, helped me pack up, put me on a plane, and then he drove across the country alone. In the dead of winter. His reward upon his return to Toronto? His sickly (unhappy) little girl. I had been too sick to make the cross-country trip with Dad, a trip that only months earlier had ushered in exciting new opportunities and adventures. My time among the mountains was over.

How was my solo plane ride back to Toronto? Terrible. I was sky high above clouds and mountains, but inside I felt like I was walking into the deepest and darkest valley of my life. I had never felt such heartbreak and defeat. Settled back in Toronto and under the watchful and fearful eyes of my parents, my well-being and vitality slipped further and further from me. In simplest terms, I felt like I was waiting to die. Heading back to my parents' home was a return to another earlier nightmare. No motherhood. No marriage. No men. And now? No mountains.

I was not utterly self-absorbed about my defeat. Although I will admit chronic illness invites selfish thinking. While I waited for surgery and settled back into the routine of living with my parents, I noticed family constellations had changed. There was something afoot in my parents' marriage, a shifting I had sensed over the Christmas holidays, three months earlier, but couldn't quite put my finger on at the time. Mom and Dad were now sleeping in separate bedrooms, a discreet but new development. There was also a sharp tension in the house that neither Christmas cheer then or my presence now could lessen. Nothing covered up the loud silences echoing through my parents' 33-year-old marriage. I watched sadly, and as if in slow motion, my parents' relationship become an empty shell of what it once had been. Today I realize that I had hoped my return to Toronto would rejuvenate their marriage and make Mom and Dad fall in love again. You know, like how a baby is supposed to make an unhappy marriage happy! This "baby" just happened to live in the basement and be 23 years old! Life has a razor-sharp sense of humour at times. I also believe my church-going years paid off as I watched my parents drift apart. I reached for hope and faith and found both.

It was that hope and faith that inspired me to ask myself whether my body had in fact betrayed me. The more I thought about it, the more I realized that it was my dreams that were betraying me, not my body. I had been given this body at birth and my body was the hand I had been dealt. Deal with it, Melody! Each of us must play the cards we are dealt, the best way we can. As the weeks of basement-living and surgery-waiting unfolded, I began to celebrate that I was alive. As long as my kidneys and I kept kicking, I realized I still had a chance to find and chase new dreams. I was grateful that I still had a chance to reach as high as any mountain. Sure, my health had pushed me into a valley, but I started to rebuild a new map. I wanted a life with lots of music, mischief, and maybe some men too!

Men throughout my life have remained both a fascination and a mystery to me. Take my father, for example. He was my primary and first example of what and whom a man is and is not. Dad was the framework by which I judged all men. I dated and married good men, and raised a great son, in large part because my father modelled goodness. He showed me how to treat others and, more importantly (especially for a woman) how to expect to be treated. Thanks to Dad's modelling, I expected to be treated well and preferably adored and cherished!

Dad was a decent, good man. And he was also a painful mystery. A man who'd been loving, loyal, kind, thoughtful, encouraging, intelligent, and caring. But the same man who had decided to leave my mother. To walk out on his wife and grown children, which is exactly what he did in 1989. Dad was 66 years old at the time and I was 33. He chose to end his 43-year-old marriage and I don't know what possessed him to do such a thing. Dad explained nothing, apologized for nothing.

I was one of the people who "hated" him for leaving. I carried that pain in my heart for a long time. My loyalty and love for my mother demanded anger and outrage. We were all so hurt. How could he? How could he dare leave our family? Was there really nothing that could be done to salvage their relationship? Apparently not. Dad eventually remarried. Pat was a lovely woman, and they clearly adored each other. Dad was destined to have a short life and I am grateful he had the opportunity to be loved first by my mother and us, and later (and lastly) by his second wife, Pat.

Dad did eventually reconcile with my brothers and me as best he could, but soon our relationship with him had a new focus: Dad was diagnosed with prostate cancer. Given his age (Dad was in his mid-seventies), the options for treatment were surgery or hormone therapy. In consultation with his doctors and his new wife, estrogen therapy was chosen as the best path forward. As I watched Dad go through his dark night of the soul, we grew closer although not quite in the way you'd expect. One of the side effects of hormone therapy is hot flashes. I was in my 40s at the time and going through perimenopause so Dad and I would share hot-flash and night-sweat stories! It felt good to laugh during such a sad and stressful time. I have yet to meet anyone whose father had hot flashes, but the times they are a-changin'.

Dad continued living life on his terms until May 2000. He witnessed a new millennium dawn and for that I am grateful since shortly thereafter Dad was eventually admitted to hospital. There was no treatment to be done. Dad asked to go home. Shamus and I accompanied Dad home while Pat, his wife, waited at their condo. It was only once Dad was on a gurney, attached to oxygen, and accompanied by two paramedics, that we noticed the condo elevators (all of them) were out of order. Unbelievable. Shamus suggested Dad be carried up 18 floors. Oddly enough, the paramedics didn't think that was a great idea. Plus, Dad's oxygen tank was almost empty. We were forced to take Dad back to the hospital. To his room and the same bed. I suppose we all should have felt grateful for that small mercy. He didn't return home, but at least he was returned to the same hospital room. How many have had to suffer and face death alone while on a gurney parked inside a hallway?

Our family was present and attentive as Dad prepared to leave us. From his hospital bed, Dad made a point of remembering and honouring Mom's birthday as best he could. I suppose on some level Dad was asking for, and possibly receiving, forgiveness from his former wife and my beautiful mother. Dad knew that I had marital difficulties. Between discussions about hot flashes, I confided that I was still not clear whether to stay or leave Bob, Lauren's father. I also confessed that I knew I was modelling to my daughter, and my son, what to expect in a relationship and marriage, and I wasn't liking the lesson I was teaching.

One day Dad called me to his bedside. He asked me if I thought $40,000 would help me buy a house. Did I want to move out with Lauren and figure my life out? I squeezed his hand and through tears, assured Dad that he and I would buy a house when the time was right. My father unconditionally loved me. Despite me pulling back my own love from him, when I was angry and hurt, I realize that my dad worked to deepen his love for me. He knew I was angry about him divorcing my mother but he seemed to know that I would return to him in time and with love. That's parenthood, not for sissies or the shallow and faint of heart.

Dad had helped me heal my broken heart when I left Calgary in defeat. I knew that when he died, I would experience a different kind of heartbreak, a deeper type of unfolding, a deeper wound that only time would heal. To this day, I am grateful I made the conscious choice to stay with Dad as he started the slow, hard process of leaving us, of dying actively and leaving the aftermath of his absence. I am so grateful to have been with my dad when he died. What a precious gift.

I have never been afraid of dying and certainly watching my dad pass from this life to the next assured me that there is nothing to be afraid of. Death was so peaceful for him. Dad called his dying his "graduation." Before he breathed his last breath, he assured me that I would be all right.

He patted my hand and smiled. I like to think he was remembering his trip to the mountains with me.

Dad always brought me home, home to Toronto, home to myself. He helped me see that I was more than "damaged goods" or the calculation of my biggest failures. Dad, in his dying, reminded me how to dream again. What a blessing to help Dad finally feel at ease in his life and with the legacy he was leaving behind. I love you, Dad.

Chapter 6

Wounded with Wisdom

Across the street from where my parents lived there was a family from Ireland. There were six kids, five boys and one girl. Unbeknownst to me, the youngest brother had a crush on me for many years. I would often see Adrian, the youngest brother, when I was out on my daily walks. I was newly returned from Calgary, still healing physically and emotionally. After months of nodding and smiling at one another, we finally chatted. The conversation connection? Talking about his car, a bright blue Camaro with a T-bar roof. It was a nice car.

Adrian was six years younger than I, so I never overanalyzed our friendship. How could a young man be interested in an older lady like me? I even tried to set him up with one of my friends, but Adrian had his eyes, and his heart, set only on me. His visits were a welcome reprieve from my hours of lying on the couch, exhausted and frustrated by kidney disease. Adrian seemed decades healthier than I. He had so much energy and good humour! I was often perplexed by what he saw in me since I was sickly, tired, and still pretty miserable about being back in Toronto! And don't forget that six-year age difference! I was pushing 25 at the time. Oh, to be so young and foolish.

Adrian and I moved in together within the year. We rented his older brother's two-bedroom condo, a lovely sun-filled space that was about a five-minute drive from both our parents. I was working by then, grateful to be feeling well enough to contribute to our lives financially. My hours working as a bank teller were long. Standing on my feet all day made for evenings and weekends marked by exhaustion. Yet I was grateful to have energy, to be earning money again, and to have attracted a new life and direction. Living so close, visiting Mom and Dad was easy and convenient, especially since Adrian worked shiftwork as a police officer. I always had plenty of time and freedom to pop over and see my parents.

We enjoyed our lives. We both had jobs we liked and things seemed to be going fine. That autumn the unbelievable happened: I found out I was pregnant! That's right. The so-called infertile woman was with child! Everyone was shocked, especially me. The news fell from the sky like a miracle. Pregnancy was not supposed to be medically possible for me and I still carried that wounded and shattered 17-year-old girl within me. I'd never forgotten how I'd been told, cruelly and without mercy, that I'd never have a family of my own. A miracle doesn't make life perfect, though. A miracle baby didn't erase the fact that neither Adrian nor I were ready for parenthood.

Adrian and I had been together for only a little over a year. Our relationship was still developing. Having a child would certainly muddy the waters. I was 25 and Adrian was 19. We were young and certainly believed we were in love. But being in love and being parents are two very different sets of rules and expectations.

The first appointment I had with my nephrologist (kidney specialist) after I found out I was pregnant was tough. He told me I only had a 50 percent chance of carrying the baby to term. But you know what? Fifty percent is a whole lot better than zero chance. I knew that if God meant for me to have this miracle baby, I would. And I planned on both mother and baby being healthy and happy.

Despite my prayers and intentions, our lives still went into a tailspin. As a couple, we'd talked about the future but in a one-two-three sort of format: get married, buy a house, save up money, then maybe try for a baby. When I first told Adrian I was pregnant, he'd been out drinking with the boys the night before. I am certain his hangover evaporated through sheer adrenaline and panic alone when I delivered what I thought was happy news. I suppose I could have waited to tell Adrian the news face-to-face but I'd been so excited that I called him from the clinic, woke him up, and pretty much screamed, "I'm pregnant!" Adrian, to his credit, tried his best. I could tell he was horrifically hungover while receiving the biggest news of his life so far. And he wasn't even 20 years old.

As a couple we talked about what we would do with this news, the pros and cons of getting married. Because of Adrian's strong Irish-Catholic faith, there was no way we could just live together indefinitely without getting married, especially with a baby on the way. I could tell caring for a baby was not the first big adult step Adrian had expected to stumble over. His life was shaping up in ways he had never fathomed. My dreams had not changed. I wanted a family, a house and a white picket fence. Could our dreams merge and build something even more beautiful? Being a true romantic, I thought my life was occurring in a book or movie. This man wanted to marry me because as far as Adrian was concerned, getting married was "the right thing" to do.

That should have been my first red flag, Adrian's feeling of begrudging obligation versus my sense of picture-perfect destiny. My entire life I had felt as if I was damaged goods so I naturally concluded that if I didn't take him up on his marriage proposal, I'd never have a chance at happiness again. Of course, we would get married, I told myself. We should get married, I whispered to myself too. Unfortunately, real life is neither a book nor a movie. You have to work hard for a happy ending.

Almost exactly a year after moving in together, we planned a fall wedding. A couple of days before we were to get married, I was out walking with my mom. We talked about how I was agreeing to spend the rest of my life with this young man. I suddenly began to sob. Not because Adrian was such a bad person, because he certainly was not, but I was so torn. My dream was here but at what cost? I did not want to feel like I was getting married only because I was expecting a baby. Mom and I continued on our walk, silent. The show must go on, right? Mom assured me that I did not have to get married. I could decide to stay at home and she and my dad would help me raise the baby.

We married on a Wednesday in my brother's living room. David and his partner, Diane, were our witnesses. Then it was back to my parents' home for dinner. Not a very auspicious occasion. Weddings tend to be joyful and fun but our gathering felt officious and solemn. The main course was beef heart, a bloody ode to love, I suppose. My mom was famous, or infamous, for cooking obscure things. There was no alcohol to toast the newlyweds. We all needed to go to work the next day. Again, there was little joy or laughter. Thus, began married life. Nothing changed. We lived in the same condo, went to the same jobs. The biggest difference? There was a baby coming.

Despite the lack-lustre engagement (four weeks) and wedding ceremony (beef heart), I felt physically great while I was pregnant. I often wondered whether I was benefiting from the baby's kidneys. I felt so good that I was able to maintain my full-time job right up until I was six months pregnant. But I did worry that the strain between me and Adrian would begin affecting the baby. To soothe my nerves and inspire more joy in my life, I regularly played the piano at my parents' house.

There were lots of appointments and tests. The stakes and the risks were so high. I was admitted to hospital in mid-January even though the baby was not due until April. Doctors and specialists wanted to keep a closer eye on me by taking daily blood tests, more frequent ultrasounds, and plenty of stress tests. I spent most of my time reading, knitting, crocheting, and waiting. Every day I walked down to the NICU (Neonatal Intensive Care Unit) to look at the preemies, knowing that my baby would be admitted into the unit within weeks. I came to love the look of the preemies. They were so small and wrinkled, like plucked chickens, but so adorable and cute too.

My mom visited every day despite having broken her hip three months earlier after being pushed at the local skating rink. Mom would hop on the subway and come down to Women's College Hospital. She would arrive after her day as an administrative assistant with the North York Board of Education and spend a couple of hours with me. She walked with a cane so I could always hear her coming. We would have dinner together. Mom could always tell when I had just been given a blood transfusion. My feet would be pink, warm, and poking out from under my hospital blanket.

Blood transfusions made my body, not just my feet, hum happily and healthily. The impact of fresh blood on my system always reminded me of how below average I operated on normal days. Without a fresh blood transfusion, my feet and hands were colourless, sore, and stone cold. (Yes, I sound a bit like Dracula.)

Adrian and I had had some discussions about what we might name our baby. Since Adrian had been born in Ireland, I very much wanted to carry on the Gaelic tradition. I loved names like Aiden as well as Daniel, which ended up being the baby's middle name. One day, Adrian came into my room very excited. He asked what I thought of the name "Shamus." I said, "What kind of a name is 'Shamus'?" He told me it was very popular back home. I assured him that we were no longer back home, so forget about it!

As it turns out, "Shamus" is Gaelic for "James," and there is somewhat of a lineage of James men in my family. My paternal grandfather was Jakob, which is Germanic for James. My third brother was James, but nicknamed Jay. (Jay went on to name his son, my nephew, Jamie). And the newest addition to the James men? My Gaelic James, my Shamus.

Not half as important, of course, as Shamus's naming but here's another Gaelic twist. My doctors' names were James (obstetrician) and Daniel (nephrologist), my two favourite male names attached to two of my favourite doctors. And I know legions of doctors! If you're wondering, of course Daniel is an Irish name. Where'd you think the song "Danny Boy" came from? And "Danny Boy," by the way, is one of my favourite pieces to play. Again, it's amazing how things work out.

Adrian and I were reasonable people so we decided that should our baby be a girl, we would definitely not name her Shamus! Even Irish charm wouldn't allow for that.

The month I spent in hospital was comfortable. I had a private room, my own bathroom, and was allowed to walk the halls if I had the energy. I would talk to my baby inside me. I'd assure the baby that we were going to be just fine. A highlight of my stay in hospital was having a weekend pass to go back to our condo in Scarborough, visit my family, and pretend that life, and my pregnancy, were normal.

My official due date was April 5th but, as expected, my baby came early. On February 10th, the doctors announced that the baby's growth was beginning to slow. It was time to meet our baby. A caesarian was scheduled for the next day. There was no negotiating. Adrian was scheduled to work that day and no matter how much I begged the doctors for a one-day delay, they were adamant: the time to deliver the baby was tomorrow, February 11th, making our baby 10 weeks premature. The day I had waited for my whole life was about to happen. By end of day tomorrow, I would be a mother.

There were lots of emotions that night. Excitement mingled with fear. What if the baby was lacking in some way? What if the worst happened and my baby died? Despite the fear, I was certain within my heart that my baby would be small but mighty. All three of us would find a way to one another, so we did.

Adrian accompanied me to the operating room just before 3:00 pm. By the time Adrian reappeared in the operating room, he was capped and gowned, and I was fully draped. I could not see anything below my chest, which was fine with me. I only wanted to know that my baby was healthy and finally here with us. The caesarian went smoothly, or so I am told. Other than feeling a little pressure, I had no idea what was going on, and felt startled when the nurse announced that I'd delivered a son. A boy, just like I had guessed. Mother's intuition? Perhaps.

At 3:45 pm on February 11th, 1982, Shamus Daniel Fynes was born. Shamus weighed in at two pounds, seven ounces. Barely 1100 grams. His safe arrival made one of my lifelong dreams come true. I was now a mother.

Because he was born so early and was so fragile, I was not able to see my son. Shamus was whisked away almost immediately to the nearby incubator. His incubation was good news. Shamus had passed all the Apgar benchmarks that measured a newborn's skin colour, heartbeat, breathing, as well as reflexes and muscle tone. My son was small, but he was mighty too.

Adrian did get to see Shamus very briefly, a tender blessing considering the man had to rush off to work shortly after his son was born! I cannot even imagine how he stayed focused on his police nightshift. Maybe he told his partner? I am almost sure there were no cigars or celebratory beers after work, especially considering his shift ended at 7:00 a.m.

When my mom arrived at the hospital, my doctor took a shine to her. In his deep Scottish brogue, he informed my nurse there was an "anxious gran here who would love to see her new grandson." Even my mom saw Shamus before I did! I do not know for sure who was the first person to hold my beautiful, small boy. I am guessing it was a nurse, but I like to think it was my mom. I was just so happy knowing that my baby was alive and healthy that whoever held my son first didn't matter. Almost didn't matter. Almost.

I ached to hold my son, my precious miracle. As that first night wore on, I asked the nurse to wheel me down to the preemie ward so I could meet my son. I was told firmly but kindly that I'd have to wait until the next day. The nurse patted my shoulder. "Your husband will be here tomorrow, and he can take you." Sure enough, Adrian brought a wheelchair and pushed me down to the NICU (Neonatal Intensive Care Unit) to see our son. There Shamus was, naked in an incubator. He was jaundiced and being treated with phototherapy, so his tiny, tiny eyes were blindfolded. His earlobes were paper thin and had been folded forward so the tape holding the blindfold would stick. I was concerned his ears would be disfigured for life! Little did I know that his earlobes were so fragile and malleable that they could be easily reshaped back into perfection. I breathed a sigh of relief and gazed at my son, still aching to hold him.

I stayed in hospital for just over a week and saw as much of Shamus as I could. He was so small and so adorable. Still, I was not able to hold him. He needed to be in the incubator full-time. He breathed perfectly, small but mighty breaths. I could reach my hand in and rub his back. Every time I saw him, my heart sang. I said a silent prayer of thanks to God for making my dream come true.

One thing Shamus was not able to do was suckle so he was fed with a feeding tube that went up his nose and straight into his stomach. When they poured formula into the feeling tube, a nurse would simultaneously put a tiny Q-Tip into his mouth. The medical team wanted Shamus to associate suckling with food. Obviously if I couldn't hold my baby, I sure wasn't able to nurse him. Despite being assured that my baby was healthy and getting stronger, Shamus looked wounded with all the tubes and tape. He was alone and encased in a plastic shell. There were times when my gratitude and relief unravelled into fear and panic. All I wanted was to be able to take Shamus home with me.

Besides the feeding tube and electrodes that monitored his heart rate and breathing, there were daily blood tests. Just like when he was born, the nurses pricked his heel to get a drop of blood. One day while visiting Shamus, a nurse came in to do that day's blood test. Shamus was naked as usual and promptly peed all over her hand. The nurse and I laughed. She quipped that she deserved the pee because he had been through so much and she was always poking him.

Once I was released from hospital and forced to leave Shamus behind, I made the daily trek downtown to see him. How could I not? My baby was there with strangers looking after him. They were the right people for the job, but he was my/our baby. One day, about six weeks after I'd been discharged from the hospital, the nurse asked if I had had a chance to hold Shamus yet. I could only shake my head. She handed me this little blue bundle, my child. There was nothing to him. Shamus had gained weight, but he was still a lightweight. What he weighed didn't matter in that moment. I was finally holding my son. What a feeling, such happiness, joy, gratitude.

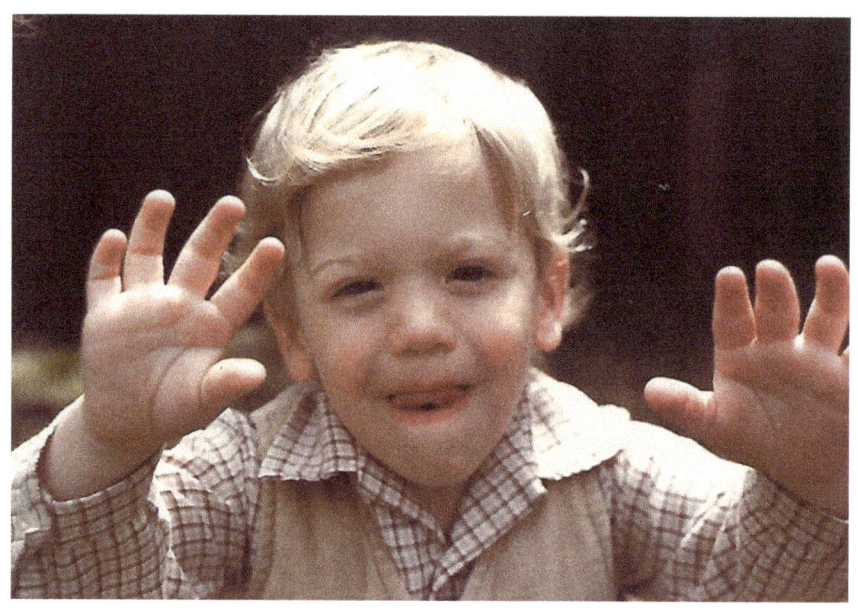

Shamus as a little boy (2), 1984

As the Easter weekend approached and Shamus was approaching five pounds, the doctors said we could take our beautiful boy home. Oh, happy day. Shamus was eight weeks old when he finally came home to us. We would finally be a family, together and reunited, in our home sweet home.

Shamus completely changed my life. And, six years later, my daughter Lauren would complete my life. Both my children have taught me much, and the beginning of my education definitely started with the arrival of my first born. I learned many lessons because of Shamus. One of the hardest was learning that dreams can come true, but there is usually a price to pay for that joy.

Not long after Shamus was home, Adrian and I decided to buy a house. We ended up getting a two-storey, semi-detached house in Oshawa, a suburb just east of Toronto. Our friends and family thought we were moving to the moon. By the time we moved in, Shamus was a healthy and happy 15-month bundle of energy. And I was in end-stage renal failure. Every day was a struggle.

Fortunately, Shamus was a great sleeper. Most nights he slept 12 hours and went down for naps at least twice a day. When he slept, I slept. I truly believe my sweet baby boy knew his mama needed the sleep so she could function another day. And another medical procedure, this time surgery. After years of waiting, a date was set for my kidney transplant. My brother Tim, and my donor, and I had to wait another 23 days. Those weeks were the longest and most stressful of my life. My biggest concern was for my brother. I knew I could always fall back on dialysis if the surgery failed, but what if something happened to Tim? My brother had a lovely wife, a young daughter, a beautiful life.

I had a young family too, but what was my choice? My body was shutting down. Shamus was 21 months old when I left him so I could return to hospital. The date was November 7th, 1983.

Once Tim and I were formally checked in and about to face a battery of tests, doctors told us that the surgery still might be cancelled, even at the last minute, if tests showed we were not a match. (Or if Tim suddenly changed his mind, which I knew he wouldn't.)

When the morning came, I knew I had a fever. Not good. Obviously, I pretended that all was fine, but Mom knew. Nurses, like mothers, are rarely fooled. I was given a cool compress and told not to worry. I was having a slight reaction to the anti-rejection medication. One of my many worst-case scenarios was that the doctors would cancel the surgery, but Tim would already be sedated. Worse than that? The surgery would be cancelled and Tim would already be cut open. I am a creative worrier!

With my fever under control, I was rolled into surgery. I asked every person who came near me if my brother was okay. Had his surgery started? Was everything going according to plan? Being put under was likely a relief not just for me but for the nurses and doctors. I could ask no more questions. I worried no more as my lights went out. A miracle happened while I was "sleeping." When I woke up in the recovery room, I was a different person; I knew immediately that I felt better! I could tell that my general malaise was dissipating. In only a couple of hours, my life was changed.

After confirming that Tim was okay, I was taken back to my room where my mom, barely recognizable in her personal protective equipment (PPE), waited to greet me. I was highly susceptible to infection in those first few days. I assured Mom that I was feeling so much better, the best-ever really, but I knew by the way she patted my hand that she thought the drugs were doing all the talking.

The surgeons told me what I could already feel inside my body: Tim's kidney had begun working as soon as it was hooked up to my system. The transplant was a good match and a successful surgery. So far so good.

Every day my creatinine, a blood waste product that measures kidney function, decreased. A normal and healthy creatinine level is between 80 to 120. Before surgery, creatinine was an unimpressive (and unhealthy) 892. Only seven days after the transplant, my level had dropped to below 200, truly a miracle. Within two weeks of the transplant, I was back at home and getting back into my usual routine: spending time with Adrian, Shamus, and my parents. I was running the household and feeling like I was on top of the world. But there's a price for joy.

Unfortunately, the surgery for the donor, for Tim, was much more invasive. Back in 1983 surgeons were drastic in their cutting. Incisions were made across the front and back of the abdomen. Muscles and flesh were severed. One of the biggest differences between the two surgeries is that the recipient goes under the knife sick and emerges a new, strong person. The donor goes in healthy, undergoes major surgery, and wakes up facing a long and hard recovery process. Tim, like all donors, was doing such a selfless thing by giving new life to another. His reward? Pain and suffering. This discrepancy seems incredibly unfair to me and still causes me to shake my head at the cruelty of it all. I remember Tim sharing how he measured his recovery post-surgery: by how long and how far he could walk. My brother celebrated his waddle-and-walk journey across University Avenue, a major street in downtown Toronto with more than six lanes of traffic. It took my brother six weeks to have the strength and speed to cross on one light. Six weeks to regain the mobility to walk across the street. Thank you, Tim. Thank you for being strong and patient. And thank you for gifting me a new life.

Chapter 7

In My Heart: David, Jay and Tim

We all know on some level that life is fragile.
Not only have I lived through illness and surgery, but I have lived through watching the people I love die. Some deaths are understandable. After a certain age our parents' deaths are not unexpected although their passing remains painful and life changing. But whether you're young or old, you never think about your siblings dying. A brother or sister is considered a peer; if you're lucky, a friend and confidant. The natural order of things is that children outlive their parents. If you've ever been forced to watch a parent bury their child, you know there's a level of sadness and devastation that's unnatural. I can't imagine the grief that any parent feels, especially a mother, but sadly I can imagine the emotional and familial wreckage better than most.

One beautiful and warm evening in June 1984, my brother David and his partner, Diane, attended a Blue Jays baseball game. David was 37 years old. After the game the couple participated in a fundraising relay sponsored by David's work. While out on the course alone, running his leg of the race, David collapsed on the sidewalk. We estimate he was alone and helpless for at least 15 minutes. David had suffered a massive heart attack and within hours of his collapse, my life-loving, laughing, and joking big brother was gone.

When I heard the news, all I remember thinking was that there was no way I would ever see David again. I was devastated knowing that I'd never be able to enjoy my brother's company or meet him for some after-work fun. David's death left me bereft. How could someone as big-hearted and loving as David have their heart betray them? I couldn't believe death could strike so suddenly and cruelly, especially since when David was taken, he was once again giving back to others. He died while running a race for charity; none of the news seemed real or fair. David was a father and had two little girls to raise. How could he be dead?

Shortly after David's death, we were surprised to learn that my brother had signed his organ donor card. Years earlier, David and Diane had had the awkward conversation about final wishes and David had been explicit: he wanted to donate as many organs (e.g., kidneys, heart, lungs) and as much tissue as possible (e.g., skin, valves, bone). In the end David's major organs stayed with him. His organs had been deprived of oxygen too long to remain viable for another soul(s), but David was able to offer the gift of sight, his corneas, to two visually-impaired strangers. David brought light and joy back into the lives of two people just as our lives dimmed and saddened with the loss of him. Life is simply too perfect to be fair, isn't it?

Since I did not have much experience with funerals, I made the decision not to attend the visitation. The last thing I wanted to see was David lying in a coffin. I did go to the funeral. The funeral was full and loving, but the pain in my heart was unbearable. I wept through the entire service. No amount of comforting made me feel better or less alone.

We were able to stay in touch with Diane after David's death, but she needed to get on with her life. I believe all of us were painful reminders of the life that had been ripped away from her. Diane eventually married and gave birth to two beautiful boys. Today, after many years apart, all of us have reconnected, and for that I am extremely grateful. Diane represents a bridge back to David that helps keep him alive in our hearts and family stories.

I can't imagine the pain my parents suffered, having to live through David's death and then forced to watch as his young girls grew up without their father. I was 27, a full decade younger than David when he died. It wasn't until I rolled up on 37 myself that I realized just how young my brother had been when he was taken from us. Now that my own son is above and beyond the age of 37, I understand even more deeply how David's life was stolen from him and us.

Death is unkind on so many levels. Life ends but life does not stop. David was gone but our lives continued to spin forward, whether we liked it or not. (I didn't.) I remember wondering how people could go about their regular routines when our world was so drastically changed. Logically I knew the death of my brother had no impact on most people but his sudden and permanent absence reminded me of Skeeter Davis' song "The End of the World":

"Why does the sun go on shining?
Why does the sea rush to shore?
Don't they know it's the end of the world?"

In the days and weeks following David's death, there was plenty of family time. We'd planned the service together while holding each other up as much as possible. Devastation was everywhere. And once the service was over, and all the guests were gone and all the funeral sandwiches were eaten, we faced a life that would never be the same. A life without David in it. We all went back to whatever we had been doing but there was now a huge hole, a massive wound, in our world. I wondered how we'd ever be the same. Answer: we wouldn't be. But life would go on.

Fast forward to 2015. David has been lost to us for 31 years. Both of our parents are gone. Dad in 2000 and Mom following 11 years later. Dad died while spring transformed into summer. Mom died in the brightness of summer. How much can a family endure? A lot, it seems. Perhaps it's our blessing and burden as humans; we can endure suffering and heartbreak again and again. One brother dead, both parents gone. My primary family decimated down to me and my two remaining big brothers.

And then? More news, more loss. That Saturday January morning in 2015 a moment in time seared into my memory. A phone call signifying the start of a new year and the beginning of another heartbreaking loss for me and our family. The nightmare kicked off with a phone call from Stratford, where Jay and his family lived. On the other end was my sister-in-law. She calmly told me that Jay had died in his sleep the night before. He'd gone to bed early, saying he wasn't feeling well.

Jay went to bed but my big brother never woke up. He was gone. Suddenly and without pain. Just like David. Jay was 62 when he died. He'd been seeing a cardiologist for months since he knew heart disease ran in our family. Jay had been as preventative as he could, always acutely aware that his brother had died young and from a heart attack. Now Jay was gone, stolen away by the same cruel and insatiable thief. When David died, I had been a young wife and mother. I had grieved with my parents. I had been hugged by my brothers. With Jay's death, there were no parents to lean on. Mom and Dad, thank goodness, were spared burying another son. I was 58 when Jay died. I was divorced, a mother for the second time, had no parents to grieve with or comfort. I muddled through my grief the best way I could. The feeling of unreality was, once again, overwhelming. His death could not be true. Jay was my closest sibling in age. We were in touch with each other more than with Tim. We understood each other and were able to communicate well and warmly. Jay simply could not be gone. I held the phone, sobbing over and over again, "No, no, no!"

Jay left behind four lovely kids, a lifelong partner, and three grandchildren. These were delights in his life he'd discussed with me over lunch less than a month before his death. We'd shared a meal on New Year's Eve day, a perfect start to a happy and healthy New Year. Or so we thought. Jay and I had happily chatted about our kids and how to best support them as they managed their moods, choices, and mental well-being. We both agreed that parenting was hard but satisfying work. Being a parent was our life's calling. We felt grateful knowing our purpose in life. I assured Jay that 2015 was going to be a good year for us both, for everyone we loved. I claimed that 2015 might even turn out to be a great year. In the end? Obviously, not so much. Life had other plans for Jay and his journey.

My brothers have always taken up a lot of space in my heart, there's so much love for them inside my beating chest, so it's not a surprise, I suppose, that I share their heart issues too! Twenty-five years after David died and while Jay was still alive, I woke up one night feeling a lot of pressure on my back, as if a fat cat was sleeping on top of me. No matter how hard I tried, I could not get comfortable. The discomfort would not abate.

I called the school where I worked that morning and told them I would come in after lunch since I wasn't feeling well. I assured my employer, and my concerned daughter, that all I needed was some extra sleep. When I finally showed up at work, a colleague urged me to visit my doctor. Her husband had had a heart attack and my symptoms, albeit appearing mild, were alarmingly similar to what her husband had experienced before going into full cardiac arrest. I took her advice and that afternoon casually drove myself to the hospital after calling my GP as well as the transplant clinic. I was so confident that nothing was seriously wrong that I felt guilty for even taking up space at the ER. But I was given a bed, had blood taken, and was offered oxygen, which immediately alleviated the pressure in my chest. Alarm bells slowly started to chime within me.

"So, you've had a heart attack," the young resident doctor announced to me and Lauren. I was so shocked by the news that I immediately burst into tears. I am not sure what I expected him to say but it was not that I had had a heart attack the night before! He looked bewildered and said, "They didn't tell you, did they? I hate it when the nurses don't inform the patient." My sickness speciality was my kidney not my heart! Another sick organ (and such an important one!) was going to be another thing I'd have to deal with now and later. And maybe for forever.

As always whenever I was admitted to hospital, I wanted to know when I could go home. The resident told me in no uncertain terms there was no way I was going home any time soon. They would need to do a coronary angiogram, a kind of X-ray to see if there was an artery blockage, narrowing, or any type of damage affecting the heart's ability to do its life-giving job.

I wracked my brain trying to think of who could rescue my car from the hospital's very expensive parking lot. Neither of my kids drive standard but then it dawned on me. Thank goodness for friends who are generous, gracious, reliable. And able to drive standard. My girlfriend and her husband not only moved my car but drove Lauren home too. I was grateful to watch some of my problems get solved despite being confined to a hospital bed.

Happily, more delights were in store. Shamus strolled in, leaving his acting rehearsal early to come and check on his mother. I am blessed with caring kids. Shamus stayed with me until I was carted away to the Cardiac Critical Care wing where I was blessed with a private room but little privacy. My kids were less than impressed when I bragged the next day that I'd taken a pee in the sink since I refused to bother a nurse for a bedpan. I am not only a private person but a clever problem-solver too! What Shamus and Lauren didn't understand, being young and 100 percent strong and healthy, was that using a bedpan made me feel powerless. If you can get up and use the bathroom by yourself, there's more dignity and control added to your hospital life.

As I admitted then, I'll admit now: I am a very independent person. I am not apologizing for being independent, merely stating a fact. Whenever I am in a medical environment, I feel like I only have two choices: stay independent and take as much control as possible or act limp and ineffective. You can imagine which approach was not my style.

I was in hospital for three days. The angiogram test showed no damage to my heart, no blockage. This was good news, indeed. I was told not to drive for two weeks. I was back at work within 10 days and chose to go back part-time. I added baby aspirin to my melange of daily pills.

I attribute my heart attack to genetic makeup, chronic grief and stress, and the amount of medication I was taking. My brothers were lighthouses, signalling the heart weaknesses we all shared. The majority of my stress and grief stemmed from three sources: my toxic romantic relationship, living with a teenager, and helping my mom recover from her stroke. Put all those factors inside a jar and shake the jar vigorously and for a long time, you're going to get a volcano. And I did. The volcano was a heart attack but thankfully, the eruption was not deadly.

Halloween 2017 brought more changes. Tim, my only surviving brother, called me out of the blue. Jay had died three years previously, David decades before. Over the years Tim and I had little contact with one another. He lived his own life and was not living in the city. Despite the distance of time and geography, I knew that if I needed something, Tim would be there for me. My brother told me he was unwell. My mind jumped immediately to cancer, but the villain was the same: a faulty heart.

Tim needed a quadruple-bypass operation. His arteries were majorly blocked, which was so shocking since Tim was Mr. Athletic. He was in ridiculously good shape. Tim was more like my dad's side of the family, all of them blessed with perfect heart health, so I had concluded (prayed) that Tim had been spared the unhealthy-heart bullet. Apparently not.

Even the Toronto surgeon was amazed by the buildup of plaque in Tim's arteries, all of it attributed to genetics not lifestyle. His heart's excellent condition was attributed to Tim's physical fitness. The surgeon told us that Tim's healthy lifestyle likely bought him an extra 20 years of life. Tim was the lucky one. The medical professionals had been able to diagnose the blockage and do something about it before he, too, succumbed to heart disease. I know for sure that David's death was heart related and can only assume the same was true for Jay. Of course, there is no way to prove my two brothers would have survived if they had been diagnosed earlier. I like to think they might have been saved but in the end, does it matter? David and Jay are gone. My heart still aches for them.

Losing a sibling is difficult and incredibly painful. Losing two is almost unbearable. I still have a hard time believing Jay is dead. David's absence still lives within me, but it's been so many years since he died. I was young when David died. Now I am wiser, older, and stronger. I am grateful that time, and love, are the great healers. Not only have my parents died, which is the expected order of things, but when siblings die it is so hard to get your head around it. At this point in time, Tim is the only person in the world who has known me all my life. My brothers were the people who had always been there, through the good times and the not-so-good times. They knew all our family stories, even the ones I never lived but I know because of their storytelling.

With two of three brothers gone, there is less grounding here in the world for me. I am grateful for the family roots I've created and grown by having my own family yet the nourishment and strength I once received from my parents and two siblings I still miss. Their impact in my life was like sunshine. When their lights were extinguished, my life grew a little darker, sadder, lonelier.

Another heart issue we all experience is heartbreak. Our hearts get broken by loss of one kind or another: the death of a loved one, the death of a significant relationship, the death of a pet, or any other sort of loss. We can either let the event rule and ruin our lives or we can be grateful for the growth that comes from being broken wide open. The loss of my brothers and parents brought pain but also taught me guidance, gratitude, and appreciation. Shamus has been guided to take care of his heart as he ages. Lauren has reported to her GP that heart issues run in the family. Both of us point out to other women that heart disease is the #1 killer in women, a fact dangerously unknown among most Canadians.

Life is too short to waste. We need to make the most of the time we have. None of us know how long we'll be here above ground. To those of you with siblings, enjoy your time with them. Siblings offer such a precious and special bond that grows love and friendship. When I look at my two children, I celebrate the friendship between them. That loving bond is part of my legacy and I am thankful to each of my brothers for teaching me the power, strength, and healing that can be found within the loving shelter of family.

Chapter 8

In My Belly: Lauren

In 1987, four years after my first transplant, I was working as a secretary in an elementary school and loving it. I was healthy enough to work full time and look after my son. My parents helped me with Shamus so much, especially by allowing us to live with them. Adrian and I had separated the year before, so life was full and busy as well as challenging. That is, until I met Bob. I was delighted to have a reliable man in my life. Meeting Bob at the community band we both belonged to (he played electric bass) was both a musical adventure and a scary stumble into dating.

Bob's grown son was living with him when we first started dating. Even though Bob and I talked about Shamus and me moving in, we needed his son to move out. In the simplest terms, until his son moved out, we could not live with Bob. There was no room, in more ways than one. Please keep in mind that I had grown up believing I would never have children because of my kidney disease. Even though I had become pregnant once, it never occurred to me that a life growing inside of me would happen again. But in the summer of 1987 I discovered that I was, in fact, pregnant again.

Like my pregnancy with Shamus, this miracle was risky too, despite my much-improved health. I felt physically terrific from Day One of my second pregnancy. There was the excitement of being pregnant and,

I believe, the physical health benefit of the baby's two healthy kidneys growing inside of me. From the moment she was conceived, my sweet baby girl Lauren was looking after me.

How much of a miracle baby was Lauren? At the time there were few kidney transplant recipients who'd been able to give birth to a healthy baby. In 1987 I was only the sixth woman in Ontario able to get, and stay, pregnant. Years later someone referred to Lauren as a miracle baby and pointed out that Bob and I, by proxy, were miracle makers; that's a title I love and appreciate especially since Lauren has brought so many miracles into my life and the lives of others.

When I told five-year-old Shamus that he was going to be a big brother and have a little brother or sister soon, Shamus very seriously informed me that his brother-to-be's name would be Andrew. Shamus also told me, equally seriously, that if it was a girl, he was leaving home and going to live with Nanny and Papa (my parents). This ultimatum was delivered while I was driving Shamus to school. It was all I could do to keep the car on the road, I was laughing so hard. Here was this five-year-old boy with a clear vision of how his life was going to unfold as well as who was going to be in his life. I told Shamus he would need to check with my parents to make potential living arrangements should a stork deliver a sister not a brother. And with that, I patted his hand and his head, and we continued on our way to school. The smile on my face never faded that day. I still chuckle at the memory. More proof that God has a delicious sense of humour.

Not long after my chat with Shamus, I remember bursting into tears one evening for no real reason. Hormones, you might say? Bob asked me what was wrong. When I was able to speak, I said that I was wondering how I could possibly have more love inside of me since my life was already so full and complete. I wanted to love this baby just as much as Shamus, but could I? Did I really have more love to give and to share? I had another miracle inside of me, but was there enough love inside of me too? Being the smart man he is, Bob assured me that everything would be fine. I was promised there would be plenty of loving room in our lives for a new beautiful life.

Once again, I was followed closely by my nephrologist (kidney doctor) and an obstetrician who specialized in high-risk pregnancies. The baby's due date was February 5th, which was also Bob's birthday! Bob beamed when he heard that news. At the time, we still didn't know if the baby was a boy or girl, and it didn't matter. As long as our baby was happy and healthy. As long as mother-and-baby continued to grow and prosper together, our small but mighty family would be fine.

December 31st, with only a little over a month before the baby's scheduled arrival date, I met with both of my doctors. That evening I'd planned on attending Tim's New Year's Eve party but the doctor I'd met with called. I was to be admitted to hospital immediately. The doctors didn't like what the tests were showing, our baby's growth seemed to be waning. I had spent enough time in hospitals over the years to know that nothing much happens on weekends and holidays, so I resented the doctor's urgency. I was confident I'd be admitted and then sit and wait.

After a lengthy conversation with the doctor, who was not my regular nephrologist but was part of the transplant team (and charming), I agreed to cancel my New Year's Eve plan and admit myself to hospital. The doctor was a kindly, older man with a trace of an Irish accent. His success in convincing me to go into hospital was a blend of his Irish charm and the Irish ability to trigger Catholic guilt. Spending days in hospital was clearly not how I wanted to ring in 1988. And I certainly did not relish a repeat of the 30 days I had been forced to spend in the hospital before Shamus was born. No one, not even a charming Irish doctor, was going to keep me away from my son for a long period of time. Plus, I believed in the health and strength of the new life getting ready to face the world. I knew this second baby was strong and therefore, so was I.

Bob had no idea our New Year's Eve plans were cancelled and that the mother of his baby was being admitted to hospital indefinitely. At the time the Irish doctor called me, Bob was at the airport picking up his two children from his previous marriage. This was long before cell phones, so I had no way of contacting Bob and telling him about the change of plans. With Dad as my chauffeur, I left a note on the front door telling Bob not to worry and to come and see me as soon as he could.

Since we had planned to have dinner with my family, I was understandably hungry when I was admitted. Remember, this was New Year's Eve. There's nothing open, especially in a hospital. Dinner that night was a stale bagel with cream cheese from a vending machine. Bob served the disaster with a smile and a shrug. We were safe and we were together. And who knew how long we'd be trapped in this room, eating junk food and feeling bored? Bob and I ended up ringing in the New Year watching Dick Clark, sharing an earbud in my hospital bed. Looking back, I realize I was happy. I was snuggled up and cared for, and each hour was an hour closer to meeting my newest miracle.

As I had feared, and similar to my pregnancy with Shamus, I was restricted to bedrest but not for as long. Two days into the New Year, I was informed a caesarian was in my immediate future. I was relieved as well as excited. Some mothers might have been frightened of delivering their baby five weeks prematurely, but my feelings were driven by gratitude that I wouldn't spend weeks in hospital! I'd be meeting my child that day. What a joy! I phoned my mom to tell them the news and Mom responded with, "Don't go anywhere until I get there." I couldn't help but laugh. I was in hospital and confined to bed rest. I truly had nowhere to go.

Fortunately, my parents and Shamus arrived in my hospital room moments before the doctor came to wheel me away to the delivery room. I expected Shamus to repeat his stork demands, wanting a brother not a sister, but instead the little guy looked at me with sadness and astonished joy. His mommy was in hospital, but she was fine. Mommy was about to introduce a new person who'd convert him into a big, dashing brother. Shamus's signature twinkling eyes made me smile and feel stronger and braver. Just as Adrian, my son's father, had done when Shamus was born, Bob scurried off to get gowned and practise tying his mask. Bob glowed with happiness and excitement.

Lauren Frances Ruth was born at 6:45 p.m., weighing in at four pounds, 12 ounces. I have it on good authority from Bob and the lovely nurses that Lauren came out waving to the world. Unlike with Shamus, who I didn't see for hours after I gave birth, I was able to admire my beautiful daughter before she was whisked away to an incubator.

Life was so good and so sweet then and in the following months and years. I had two children, a boy and a girl (what old-timers call the "million-dollar family") despite being told, when growing up, that I would never have children. The joy that I'd been promised would forever elude

Forever Grateful

me was here, twice. My children are my miracles. How can I not look out into the world and feel hope and faith that life is benevolent and kind? God blessed me with two angels, and I am grateful.

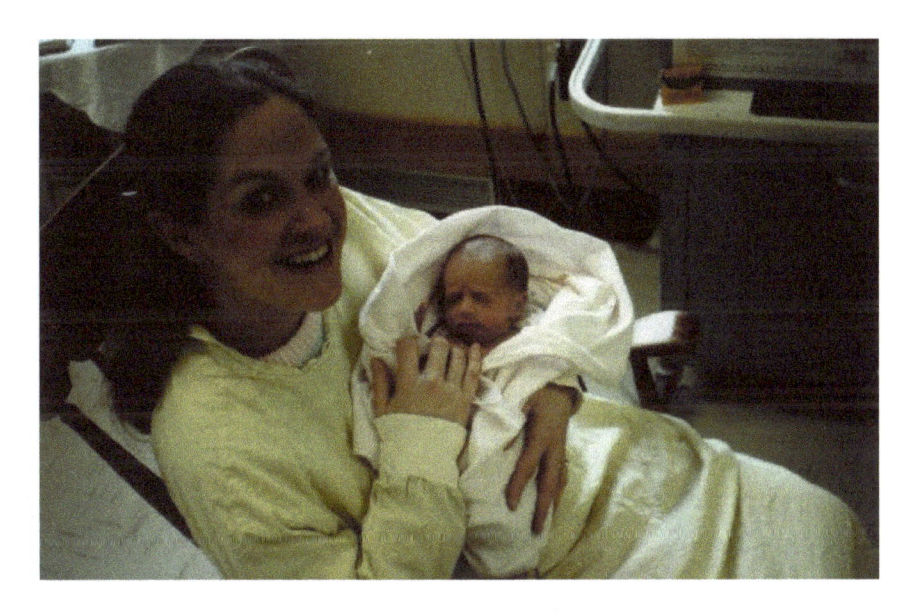

Lauren as a newborn, 1988

After Lauren's birth, there was concern that my transplanted kidney was starting to fail. My body was quickening its attempt to reject the new kidney, which would affect everything in my life including mind, body, and spirit. Hours after Lauren's birth, the decision was made to do a kidney biopsy on me. A biopsy entails inserting a needle into the kidney and removing some cells for testing. After a biopsy, you are required to spend 24 hours in bed to avoid hemorrhaging (bleeding). So, another full day in hospital was scheduled when all I wanted to do was be discharged so I could be at home with my two children and partner. Instead, this new joyful chapter in my life was delayed.

As fate would have it, the test results were inconclusive. My kidney was doing the best it could considering the shift in hormone levels post-birth. I offered to come to hospital every day in the weeks ahead to have blood work done. I wanted my medical team to release me from jail... I mean, hospital. I prayed for a solution not a sentence. My doctors agreed to release me so I escaped home, safe and sound, just two weeks after the birth of my precious baby girl.

Once we were all home and now a family of four, life settled into something of a routine. Shamus was well into his Senior Kindergarten year. I, once again, was able to experience and enjoy motherhood. Lauren was not nearly as good a sleeper as Shamus, but then again, I didn't need as much rest. Mother and daughter figured out their routines and schedules. Now that I had two children, life was busier but also more fun. With Shamus being in school full time, Lauren and I had lots of time to ourselves. We enjoyed being outside, walking the streets of the neighbourhood, visiting Mom and simply being in each other's presence. Lauren and I developed our own special language and could read each other's moods and mindsets without a word but always with a smile. Hugs at home were frequent and forever welcome. Bob was an attentive father and partner. Again, life was good. Every night I counted my blessings and expressed gratitude. I was so grateful for my health and the well-being of those I loved and cherished, especially since those loved ones were legion in number.

Since my children are almost six years apart, it was challenging finding activities that we could do together as a family. Anything that Shamus might enjoy was way beyond Lauren's interest and/or capability. And, of course, activities or interests appropriate for Lauren were certainly of no interest to Shamus. But we found a way, slowly but surely and with a few stumbles. One time we decided to take the kids to the movies and allowed Shamus to choose. We went to see "Ace Ventura: Pet Detective." Shamus thought the movie was positively hilarious. I'll only admit to feeling relieved that most of the off-colour humour was way beyond Lauren's understanding. We did eventually discover that mini-golf was a suitable and relatively enjoyable family activity! Bob had a good putting aim and I was not overly talented (or competitive). Shamus could always get the ball through the littlest holes and Lauren was an expert at shooting the ball straight through the windmill.

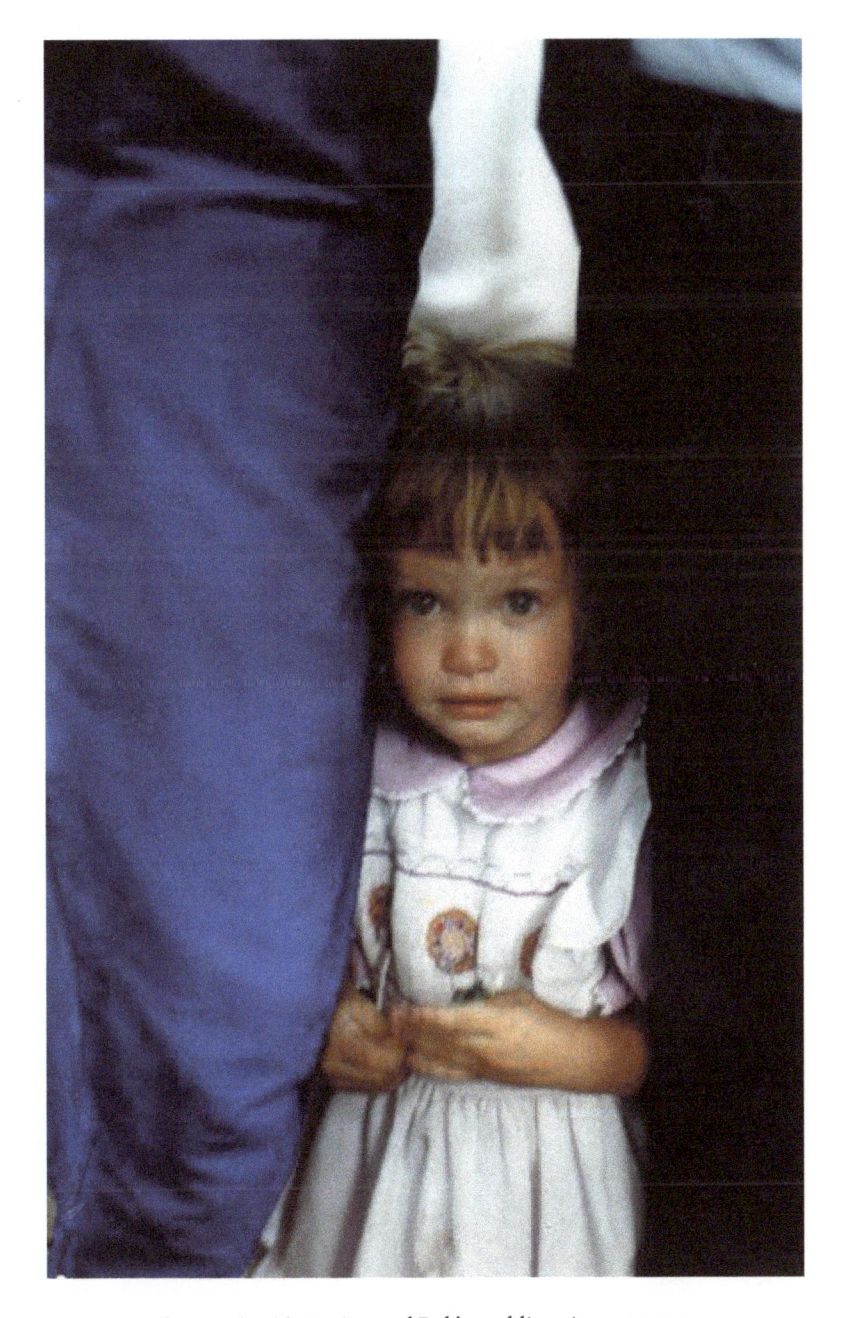

Lauren (2 1/2) at mine and Bob's wedding, August 1990

We were able to have fun at home together playing games, reading books, watching movies. Shamus often had friends over, which made the house loud and happy. We were known to bundle up and go for walks in the winter or take the kids skating at the local rink.

My gratitude for being a mother knows no bounds. Without transplantation, Shamus might have been an only child. But because of the miracle of organ donation, I have two wonderful children. Life has expanded to include two fantastic granddaughters. Again, life is good. Then and now.

Chapter 9

In My Life: My Kids Are My Joy

The thing with children is they have no choice about what happens in their lives. We all learn what we live. My kids lived the reality of their mother's fragile health. Shamus and Lauren knew that their mom was not like other moms. Most kids had parents who were so healthy that there was never a reason to think about health, well-being, and the fragility of life.

My children grew up with a mother who was "delicate." Not weak like cooked spaghetti but fragile like crystal. When your health is uncertain and volatile, divided into good days and terrible in-the-hospital days, life is different for those around you, especially your children.

Because of the uncertainly of my health, I expected my children to pull their weight around the house and to know how to do things on their own. From the time they were in Grade 2, I expected Shamus and Lauren to make their own lunches. Not a big deal by my standards, and, unlike most of their classmates, the kids seemed to enjoy the independence of making their own menus. After having worked in education for many years, I've grown appalled by the number of kids who, even when they are in high school, do not make their own lunches. They'd complain about their lunches and I'd be the grown-up who'd tell them that if they just made their own, they wouldn't complain because they'd eat what they love. My excellent advice usually fell on deaf ears.

The household talents of my children were endless. They knew how to do laundry, cook simple meals, and complete general household chores. (If you're reading this and reflecting on how lazy your kids were growing up, you might want to consider how much you never asked your kids to do). Kids can do a lot if they're motivated and praised. If they're convinced housework is grown-up work, all the better.

Both Shamus and Lauren had specific rotating chores that we set each week on our posted Chore Chart. We never wanted the kids to feel overloaded or, heaven forbid, discriminated against. There were no "gender roles" in our home when it came to chores. I was neither raising a future chauvinist nor a housewife-to-be. Shamus and Lauren don't scare easily, in large part because of my roller coaster health. They usually don't panic when faced with challenges, and they are unlikely to roar or whine about the "unfairness" of life. Life is what it is, and our job is to deal with life's lemons the best way that we can.

If we are looking for heroes in this story, I would have to say that they are my children. I dealt with illness because that was the hand I was dealt. They survived my illnesses and are better people for it. They are stronger, more flexible, deeply compassionate, and definitely capable of handling life's hard balls. Shamus and Lauren are well rounded adults with good values that lead to good decisions for themselves and others.

I was able to help my kids develop the skills to cope in a crisis. They have certainly dealt with their fair share of bad breaks and situations totally out of their control (and mine). I am grateful that my major health crises and hospital stays happened when the kids were older, Shamus 13 and Lauren seven, rather than when they were young. I'd never have wanted the kids to feel confused or abandoned because of my hospital stays. Even when they were older, it often broke my heart to leave them behind at home.

Teenagers are traditionally self-absorbed and selfish, but Shamus and Lauren were focused and attentive whenever Mom (me) had a medical crisis. Whether it was diverticulitis, appendicitis, a heart attack, or general scrapes and bruises with plenty of bleeding, my kids had learned how to react calmly and quickly in a "Mom crisis."

When I had to have my appendix out, Shamus took me to Emergency and stayed with me all day. Since he works from home full-time, he settled into my hospital room and worked from his laptop. That particular day, Lauren was supply teaching followed by teaching her private music students. Even after such a full day, once my girl was finished her work, she joined me and Shamus at the hospital until I had my surgery around midnight that night. The next morning Shamus was back and ready to drive me home. God bless my kids.

Even if I was unwell, my kids knew they could always count on me. I would be there for them even if it was from a hospital bed. I remember when I had peritonitis and was in a lot of pain. Shamus called me and wanted to know about getting Lauren a kitten for Christmas. I suggested that perhaps this wasn't the best time to talk about getting another cat. But, for him, just because I was in hospital, there was no reason not to talk about it. End result? We did get a kitten for Christmas. The kitty, "Holly," was adorable: fluffy, grey, and white. Like a dog, she'd follow us on walks. Perhaps the cat is like me, blessed with nine lives and plenty of reasons to purr and feel grateful for the kittens (kids) in our lives.

Chapter 10

Lessons from Little Ones

Shamus was a born entertainer. He was always ready with a song, joke, or dance. A real cutie, with blonde curly hair and a ready smile. But that smile was only present if I was near at hand. As a boy Shamus was always a bit concerned when his mommy was nowhere to be seen. He would become distraught, cry, and wonder aloud where his mommy was. When Shamus was going through this particularly clingy stage, I didn't understand why it bothered him so much when I left the room for a moment or, worse, tried to go to the bathroom by myself. But with time and perspective his behaviour made sense. We had spent eight weeks apart when he was first born so I'm confident that absence is seared into Shamus's DNA, as it is mine. I still feel a twinge today when I remember the pain of not holding my newborn son for almost two months. So I hold him extra tight today.

Growing up, Shamus experienced multiple episodes of "Where's Mommy?" Rarely did he receive an adequate answer. When he was just a toddler, I vanished, hidden away in a hospital room for over two weeks as I prepared for and recovered from my first kidney transplant. Just a few years later, I vanished again, multiple times. Every time his father came to pick him up for a weekend or holiday outing, I was gone. His father, Adrian, and I were living apart and in the process of divorcing.

When I informed Shamus that he and I were going to move out and live with Nanny and Papa (my parents), his one and only question was, "Can I take my bike?" The important things in life to a child.

Shamus was able to eventually take things in stride. His entertaining ways were legendary within the family. Apart from telling jokes, he did a fabulous rendition of "Danny Boy" up until he was about 10. He was so sincere as he stood and sang. Shamus looked like a character in Charlie Brown, his mouth open so wide that his face disappeared. As Shamus grew older, I told him he was destined to be a lawyer or an actor because he could so naturally speak to people whether one-on-one or to an audience. I also told him that there really was not much difference between a lawyer and an actor, except the pay grade!

When my son started dating, I was concerned about who he would choose as a spouse and life partner. Shamus and I have always had a very special relationship. For years it was just me and Shamus making our way through life and doing the best we could together. It is commonly believed that people choose partners similar to their parents. If this were true for Shamus, he would have chosen a woman who was sickly and with lifelong struggles with well-being and health. A woman who was strong and feisty but not particularly healthy.

At the time of this writing, Shamus has been married for over 10 years. He's the proud father of two magical little girls, Emma and Lily. Their mother, April, Shamus's wife and my lovely daughter-in-law, is one all-round gorgeous person. Shamus chose a spouse who is healthy, vibrant, and certainly strong, inside and out. Like his mother, April can keep up with Shamus and hold her own against our legendary entertainer. The similarities we share in personality extend to our physicality too. We're both small, petite, and brunette. In other words, April and I are great beauties. And humble to a fault.

Speaking of beautiful things, the relationship between April and my daughter is also a delight and blessing. I realize that as a mom I was within reason to wonder (worry?) about my son's romantic decisions. But it's watching the friendship between Lauren and April, and the special relationship between Auntie Lauren and her two tiny nieces, that I realize how blessed we all are to have found each other. I believe one of the reasons Lauren connects so easily with most people is because she's compassionate and always looking out for the underdog. She loves family and all animals. That love is matched by a passionate dislike for liars and those who pretend to be what they are not.

When Lauren was 18, she decided to get her first tattoo. We talked it over. She was of age and there was nothing I could do about it. The only thing I said was, "Please be safe. Go somewhere reputable where you will not get sick." She's followed that advice each and every time she's gotten a tattoo, over and over again. My beautiful daughter now has 10 tattoos, the majority are exquisite and artistic. (Yes, I have my favourites.) The body art is her decision, her choice, her body. Like the tattoos themselves, Lauren's decision-making process was well-thought out and helped inspire tattoos that are both beautiful and forever meaningful.

One of the most poignant tattoos is on her left leg. It's a lollipop with a string bean climbing up a stick. How is that well thought-out? My dad, Lauren's grandfather, known as Papa to the grandkids, used to call Lauren "Lolly" and "Lollipop." His nickname for Shamus was "String Bean." You can imagine why that tattoo is my favourite. It's a testament to Lauren's love of family, her childhood love for my dad, and her deep friendship with big brother Shamus. I wept when Lauren showed me the artist's rendition of her vision. I cried harder when Lauren told me she was getting "inked" with the lollipop-string bean image on the 10th anniversary of her grandfather's death. She's a gentle soul, kind and thoughtful.

Lauren approaches the world with so much vulnerability and openness. My protectiveness of my girl child is fierce and I often have to remind myself that both my children are strong and capable. They don't need me as much as they once did, and that's how life is supposed to unfold. For example, when Lauren first started getting her tattoos, I wanted her safe and I also demanded she not regret her (permanent) decision. I was clear about what I didn't want to hear: whining or expressions of regret.

Given all that I have had to deal with in my life, experiences totally outside of my control or preference, I have very little tolerance for people (even children) who are whiners. There is no point complaining about being stuck in traffic, gaining five pounds, or catching a cold. My reaction to whining of this low calibre is swift and immediate: I invite the offending chronic whiner to visit a dialysis unit or pop into a chemotherapy treatment centre. Harsh? Perhaps. But you're not going to hear whining and complaining inside places like that. Those sick people are too busy fighting for their lives and trying their best to make life bearable for themselves and their loved ones.

Like I said, I am often more fire than warmth, especially when people are being ridiculous. But I really do want people to have an understanding, some perspective, about their blessings in life. I like the saying about how most people have many wishes. But an unhealthy person has only one wish: to feel healthy again. I believe I've walked marathons in those shoes, so I speak freely and passionately about whining: stop!

Don't sweat the small stuff. Be like Lauren and never regret a tattoo or a decision you can't take back. Be kind and vulnerable and brave. And always remember to sing your head off like Shamus, especially if you're singing "Danny Boy."

Chapter 11

Role Model

Every summer growing up, my mom expected, and insisted, that our summer holidays include a car trip to Manitoba to visit her only sibling, her sister Ida. Mom wanted us to connect with the people and places that shaped her Western childhood. These long car trips from Toronto to Steinbach and Neepawa were during a time when air conditioning and seat belts were rare. The annual car trips to Manitoba started when Mom and Dad were in their 40s. Their passengers (hostages?), my brothers and I, were between the ages of four and 13. Being the youngest and smallest, I usually ended up stuck in the middle of the front seat between my parents or, worse, between my brothers in the back seat. Not my idea of a good time. All I wanted was to sit by the window, watching the landscape go by. The whining and fights were legendary and legion.

Every year when we returned home, Mom vowed never to car trip to Manitoba again. Yet the next summer always signalled Mom's deep desire to see her family. Mom modelled the lesson, again and again, that we need to make the most of the time we have with our loved ones. My mother had a dignified and strong depth of character and loyalty, which served her well during good times and hard times too.

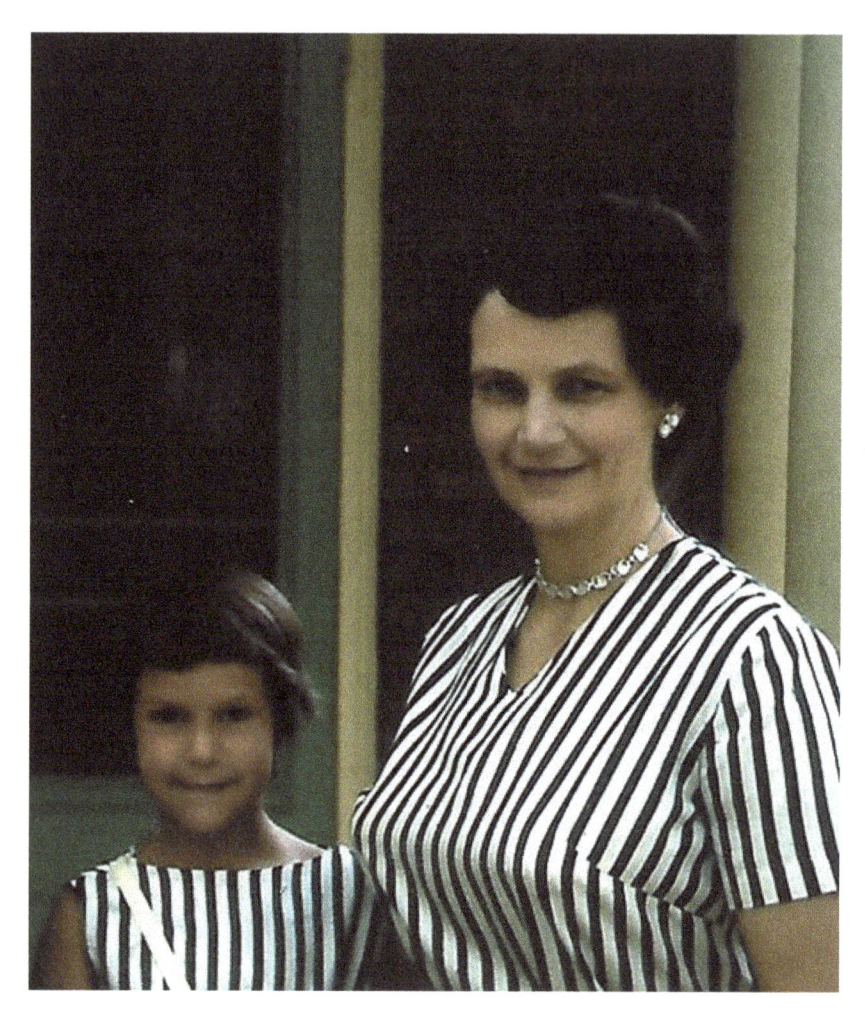

My mom and me in Peterborough, circa 1963

In 1988, four years after David's death, my dad, after 43 years of marriage, decided he was leaving our mother. Mom was to be on her own for the first time ever. She would need to make her way in the world alone. My mom was of the generation where women went from living at home to living with their husband. She had never had the opportunity or interest in living on her own and managing her own affairs. Why would she? Mom had always been taken care of, and now the world and her place in it had drastically and cruelly changed.

By the time Bob and I were getting married, Mom's sister, Ida, had died. This was 1990 and Ida had left behind her husband, my Uncle Dudley, widowed and lonely. Their daughter, Yvonne, lived near her father and she and her family helped as much as they could. But my mom recognized the suffering within her brother-in-law. They both missed Ida and they were both alone. Mom was alone through divorce, Dudley through death. Mom had lost her best friend, and in many ways, Dudley had too. I was glad when Dudley, Yvonne, and her husband decided to join us in Toronto to celebrate our nuptials. The three of them travelled from Neepawa, Manitoba, and Mom was ecstatic.

My mother had been divorced from Dad for several years and happily had the room and the mindset to host her Manitoba family. We all recognized it was a big deal for Dudley and his family to travel to the big city for our wedding. Dudley and Ida had lived their whole married life in rural Manitoba. Their lives were fairly uncomplicated, but they had always been busy. Dudley owned an implement dealership (International Harvester) before buying a chicken farm. Ida had spent her time doing charity work and keeping a warm and orderly household.

Dudley had been staying in Mom's home for mere days when he invited Mom to accompany him to Australia for six weeks. If they could survive each other for six weeks, he told her, they might consider making their relationship a permanent arrangement. In other words, Dudley was offering his former sister-in-law security and a new life, but back in Manitoba where she'd grown up. Mom was being invited to go home again.

To say that this turn of events was surprising is putting it mildly. I think Mom was shocked that anyone else would want to be with her. When Dudley first mentioned his marriage idea, she thought he was joking. Obviously, our family was flabbergasted. If Mom accepted the marriage proposal, it would mean Mom leaving me and my brothers behind in Ontario. The plot thickened. Dudley's children were my mom's niece and nephews. If she married Dudley, she'd replace a niece and three nephews with four stepchildren! My cousins would now be my stepsiblings. I had always wanted a sister, but this is not what I had in mind.

As this idea grew and seemed more and more likely to happen, that Mom would visit Australia, come home and marry Dudley, and move to Manitoba permanently, I began to realize how much my life would change. There would be no more daily conversations, no deciding to drop in for a visit, no more dropping the kids off at Mom's. It was a hard adjustment for both of us, but Mom had something really positive to look forward to. Family was always a priority for Mom. She loved her family and wanted to keep everyone together. Mom was always the one who arranged family get-togethers, including a party in February to celebrate all the winter birthdays in our family. There was Lauren in January followed by five February birthdays for Shamus, two nieces, a nephew, and Bob. We couldn't imagine life without Mom. She was the glue that kept us together. As my brothers and I had feared, once Mom was married and moved to Manitoba, Toronto family traditions stopped. No more get togethers, not much communication, and eventually everyone went their separate ways.

Looking back, I admit I was torn about the Australian trip, a kind of six-week "trial marriage" for Mom and Dudley. What would happen Down Under? What would happen once they were home? What would Toronto life look like without Mom in it? The newly anointed couple flew out Boxing Day and they wouldn't return for six weeks. Like when I was a teenager and touring overseas, singing in choir, Mom wrote me regularly. It was always a great day when I received an update on their activities. My brothers and I never ceased wondering what would happen when Mom arrived home. Would she marry Dudley? Would they hate each other in Australia? Would we be happy or sad? Or would we feel a blend of both emotions, happy that Mom was happy but sad Mom was moving away?

Once Mom was back in Toronto and Dudley had returned to Manitoba alone (for now), Mom and I went for a long walk touring Edwards Gardens in Toronto's north end. As we admired the flowers, Mom was upbeat and fresh, no longer jet lagged. She was tanned from Australian sunshine. She said the trip had been interesting, educational, and that she wished she had been able to travel more in her younger years. Our walk consisted of talking, laughing, and sometimes crying. I could tell Mom was leaning towards marriage and Manitoba. There were doubts. She wondered aloud about what Dudley would be like as a husband. Mom was 66 years old and curious if she could really start all over again with a new man, a new marriage, and a new life. Mom was contemplating marriage at the age I am now as I write this chapter. It's interesting to make some comparisons. Could I make a new start in a different place? Would I want to? Could I leave my family for a man?

Mom and I shared some common concerns. What would life be like in rural Manitoba after so many years in Toronto? In Toronto Mom had access to arts and culture like the city's renowned orchestra, live theatre, and world-famous musical productions. She was a dedicated lifelong learner and had spent years learning Hebrew. What was the likelihood of studying another language while living in rural Manitoba? Or attending the symphony?

Another big concern we both shared was if/when Mom moved to Manitoba, was she really obligated to marry Dudley? Mom would have been just as happy living together and avoiding a formal legal arrangement. Yet Mom knew the rural community well and was resigned to the fact that she would neither be welcomed nor accepted unless she was Dudley's wife. I appreciated how Mom wasn't overly concerned about the community disapproval if she chose to move to Manitoba but not marry Dudley. Mom knew who she was and was confident the community would see the quality of her character. She'd been visiting her sister Ida for years. The community could never deny that Mom was a loyal and loving woman. Despite our common concerns and fears, Mom and I knew one thing for sure: we would always be there for another. When Mom married and moved less than a year later, I knew life had changed but I also knew that Mom and I would always have each other.

Their wedding in 1991 was ominous. The wedding day was June 16th, the same day that David had died seven years earlier. Mom said she wanted to replace a sad memory with a happy one. The entire family, on both sides, had high hopes for a happy marriage and a long life for the couple. Most people would consider it odd that my mom married her sister's widowed husband. In our family we weren't shocked or deeply disturbed by the turn of events. Our lineage has plenty of "keeping it in the family" marriages. For example, my paternal grandmother was the second wife of my grandfather. When my grandfather's first wife died, Mennonite custom dictated that the widower return to the deceased wife's family and marry the next available daughter. That is how my great aunt became my grandmother. She was 19 years old, used to working outside, and loved riding horses. My great aunt (to be grandmother) grew up having zero interest in housework or having children. Yet upon the death of her older sister, she was married off and inherited children, her niece and nephews. The eldest child was less than a decade younger than their new stepmother. A difficult position for everyone involved, indeed.

Packing up Mom's boxes in Toronto and shipping them to Manitoba was bittersweet. Dozens of boxes were filled with skeins of wool for knitting and crocheting, two of my mother's favourite hobbies. My brothers and I concluded that Mom was a bit of a wool hoarder. Most people buy a single ball/skein. Not my mom. She would buy at least six, if not eight, balls depending on whether or not the wool was on sale. She bought the skeins not because she needed them or had a specific project in mind but to have lots of wool in the house "just in case." I must admit that Mom's wool hoarding came in handy many times for me. Rather than having to go out and buy wool, I would simply go to Mom's stockpile and help myself. As I helped her pack up, we had lots of laughs about her "just in case" wool hoarding. What would I do without her?

Mom moving to Manitoba was one of the hardest experiences of my life. The separation was so painful. We knew the move was a good thing for both of us, but that did not make the pain any less. I remember once sitting on the living room floor and sobbing like a little girl, missing my mom. In those first few weeks and months, I missed my mom's presence. As the years unfolded and she grew older and frailer, I missed my mother's vitality and vivaciousness.

Mom had been married to Dudley for 13 years when she had a stroke. She'd been visiting us in Toronto when her health failed her. The devastation of the stroke sentenced her to a life without knitting and crocheting. Along with the majority of her physical abilities, the stroke abruptly and cruelly stole her stockpile of joy too. After the stroke, every time I visited Mom in rural Manitoba she'd insist I bring home one or two of her still-unpacked wool boxes. Imagine that. The wool had been packaged up more than 13 years prior! Every time Mom insisted on gifting me her wool, my heart unravelled a little bit more. I flew to rural Manitoba regularly so I accumulated a lot of wool in my Toronto home(s). Funnily, just recently I donated the majority of Mom's wool to a seniors' craft group. I could feel Mom smiling down on me as I made the donation. I am no longer a wool hoarder like my mom!

The years prior to Mom's stroke and afterwards demanded we get more comfortable with being apart. We were surprised to conclude that our separation made us grow and taught us about strength, resiliency, and the importance of staying in touch. I know that I grew up a lot after Mom left and she learned a lot about herself too. The distance also changed one tradition. Before Mom moved away, neither of us made a big move or important decision without consulting the other. Once we were separated from one another, we were forced to rely more on our intuition and old-fashioned grit. I still had my mother's back and she had mine. But both of us were forced to grow stronger, wiser, and less reliant on outside advice. Neither of us had access to the other's thoughtfully explained opinions and passionate pieces of advice anymore. The Ontario-Manitoba dynamic pushed us into new roles shaped by self-reliance and self-confidence.

We continued to regularly communicate, just not every day. Saturday morning phone calls became our new ritual and something I savoured the entire weekend. During the week I was blessed to receive at least one letter from Mom. She was a much better letter writer than I and certainly diligent. Mind you, I did have two young children who needed my constant attention so writing letters back to Mom bordered on daunting to impossible.

I have been so fortunate to have such a strong and self-sufficient woman in my life. It is no wonder that I always wanted to be a mom. I had such a wonderful role model. I truly feel like I knew my mom inside out, possibly better than she knew herself. I believed that she was much more capable than she believed. Even though she had her doubts about her move to Manitoba, I knew she would handle her new life beautifully. Her determination and commitment were indomitable.

Having such a wonderful mother, friend, and role model has inspired me to be the best mother and person that I can be. My mom always had time for people, would help out where and when she could. Even when she was being robbed of her eyesight with macular degeneration (the deterioration of the macula, which is the central portion of the retina and the leading cause of vision loss in people over the age of 60), she continued to go to the local long-term care home and read to the residents once a week. She was able to read clearly by finding large print books and using a magnifying glass. Physical limitations did not deter her from helping others. Often when I visited Mom in Neepawa, we'd visit Mom's long-term care resident friends. I'd play my harp and feel proud that I was my mother's daughter.

Throughout all that she dealt with in her life, Mom's faith continued to grow and uphold her. Once she moved to Neepawa, she joined a Bible study and often led the group. Given her knowledge of the Bible, she had wisdom to share. Mom lived a very Christian life in all senses. Not in a showy way but in a quiet, understated, and authentic way. There was always a Bible close by and often a study book of some kind. I know she prayed often. Again, not in a showy way but quietly and privately. She was grateful for all she enjoyed in life and as far as I know, Mom never uttered a harsh word about anyone. Before her stroke, she'd visit us in Toronto and tell us about all the things she loved about rural Manitoba: the big sky, the peace and quiet, the assortment of birds and wild animals. She had the ability to come and go as she pleased, spend time in the kitchen baking or making jam, or going into town to volunteer and help those in need. She admitted that she loved coming back to Toronto not just because of us but it was good to be reminded there was a much bigger (and louder) world outside of small-town Manitoba. Periodically she needed to come to the city to remember that there was a bigger world.

As the years passed, no matter how often I suggested Mom carry a white cane because of her failing eyesight, the answer was always an adamant "No!" I assured her she did not need to use the cane but to consider carrying the cane around so people would know she was visually impaired. Only once did Mom admit to getting on the wrong subway and going the wrong way because of her sight. She didn't find the story funny but I did and so did the kids. Shamus and Lauren loved it when their grandmother visited Toronto and stayed with us. Mom and Lauren had to share a bed, which thankfully delighted them both.

When I was at work, Mom would do helpful things around the house like doing the laundry, tidying up, and making meals, things that made my day easier. Then there were the times we were able to get away, just the two of us, for shopping, visiting friends, or going down to Queen Street to have a shared Maple Dip doughnut and a cup of tea at Tim Horton's. If the kids were involved in anything extracurricular while Mom was visiting, she was always keen to attend. She made a point of coming to Toronto for special events such as recitals or graduations. It was important to her to be as much a part of the kids' lives as possible even though she lived far away. Mom was still their granny and she wanted Shamus and Lauren to always remember who she was and how much she loved them.

My mom was, indeed, a special lady. She had a way about her. She grew up so much as a woman, wife, and mother. Mom was always changing, especially as her children grew up and moved into their own loves and lives. She'd been a young wife to a minister, a young mother to three sons and an unwell daughter. Mom watched as two of her children underwent major surgery on the same day: my first kidney transplant, Tim's gift of life to me. Then, less than a year later, Mom was forced to bury David, her eldest child. I believe my mother's heart broke permanently that day. I can't imagine the shock and sorrow. Yet nevertheless she persevered.

To say I am in awe of my mother's strength and kindness is an understatement. She was one of the most influential forces in my life and I am grateful that force opened me and deepened me to the power of love, gratitude, perseverance, and strength. She shone a bright light and I carry that light within me. I admire that same brightness in the hearts of my children, and for that I am especially grateful. Not only was Mom an excellent role model, she made such a loving impact on her grandchildren and her friends. Mom is forever connected to me and our family. Ask anyone about Ina, my beautiful and loving mother, and they will tell you what a special lady she was.

Chapter 12

Summer from Hell

The summer of 1995.

In our family that charming period of time is lovingly known as the "Summer from Hell." Lauren was seven years old and Shamus 13. We lived in Toronto in an area known as The Beach, an upper middle-class neighbourhood in east end Toronto. Bob, Lauren's dad and the head of this (blended) family, had purchased the house in 1986 shortly after his first marriage ended. He had a job in the accounting department of Confederation Life Insurance. As far as I knew, we were comfortable but not wealthy. I felt fortunate to be at home with my children in their formative years. Since having children had been a lifelong desire for me, I most certainly wanted to be with them when they were growing up and doing their "firsts:" first steps, first words; those kinds of firsts. Having children had been my dream my whole life so I did not want to miss a moment. As with Shamus, when Lauren was born, I knew I was going to stay at home with her until my baby girl headed off to school.

I remember years earlier, when Shamus was an infant, I visited the bank where I used to work. I was chatting with some of my former clients and one of them asked me when I was coming back. They seemed surprised when I said I wasn't. When asked why, I told them that I wanted to be with my son as he grew up. The clients told me I could pay someone to do that! Clearly these people did not know me very well. Their question implied that I enjoyed their company more than my children's! I shake my head at the absurdity. I dedicated my life to my two dreams, my son and my daughter, and wouldn't change a moment of baby time for bank time. My colleagues and clients had been nice enough, but they weren't *that* nice. Their company sure couldn't compete with my babies! Raising and being with my children full time was decidedly my priority and the source of my joy and life's meaning.

Yet funnily enough, as much as I enjoyed being with my children, there came a time when I decided I needed some outside stimulation. So I decided to get a part-time job. Given the neighbourhood we lived in, I was fortunate enough to find one on nearby Queen Street in a children's clothing store. The job was fun. I was able to socialize, earn a little money, and get some great clothing for Lauren at a discounted price. There were times when payday came around and I was lucky if I made any money at all since most of my wage was spent expanding Lauren's wardrobe.

Going back to work was dependent on finding a wonderful neighbourhood caregiver, which I did. Leaving Lauren the first few times was a bit bittersweet. While I was looking forward to enjoying some adult time and socializing outside my home, I also missed spending time with my much-loved baby girl. But I knew going back to work part-time was the right decision for me, and for the kids. Lauren was able to socialize with another woman and play with other children. Meanwhile, Shamus was at school and growing more independent by the second. Healthwise, I was doing great. While I was working at the clothing store, I didn't bother taking breaks. I never sat down, stretched, or had a glass of water. I felt so good, I didn't even need to go to the bathroom! Ten years after my kidney transplant, I was thriving and filled with gratitude for the relief and freedom of good, strong health. I religiously took my medications, ate properly, drank plenty of water (at home), and always slept well. I had the sneaking suspicion my health might stabilize forever.

After about a year, I was ready for a new challenge. There was a small and independent store called "Sound City" that sold CDs and DVDs. The owner was a nice young man who took a chance on hiring an older woman who did not really have much experience. Often I was there on my own, which made it challenging to get to the bathroom. My solution was to stop drinking water while working, a habit I'd reinstated after my doctors, each and every one of them, told me water was imperative in keeping my kidneys flushed out and functioning properly.

Because I'd been feeling good for so long, I'd grown complacent about the impact of my lifestyle choices. I was working hard at home and at work, and indulging in bad habits that were the epitome of anti-kidney health. Yes, it's hard to imagine that not drinking enough water can cause terrible health consequences, but that's the reality of having kidneys that are always debating whether they are sick or spectacular! In simplest terms, I did not realize my good health was being sabotaged. My creatinine, a body waste product the kidneys filter out, was getting higher by the day. But I was not even aware of the growing toxicity inside my body. I felt fine, that is until I received the results of my blood tests months later. I had no idea that within weeks I'd have doctors descend on me, delivering yet again more bad news. Welcome to the summer from hell!

As my health quietly diminished, Confederation Life, where Bob worked, was forced into liquidation. Within the year, my husband would be out of a job. It was a devastating time for Bob as he had been employed with "Confed" for many years. He expected to retire as a celebrated accounting manager. As far as Bob was concerned, he had played "by the rules" and had lived life the way it was supposed to be lived: he graduated from high school, was successful at college, started a career, and expected his career to end with a "golden handshake." Bob had looked forward to a proud, prosperous, and joyous retirement for years. His dream, like his job, was terminated.

As we went into the spring and summer of 1995, life definitely had its stresses. There was a lot of tension in the household, but I was determined that the kids would have a good summer, including having them spend time with Mom in Manitoba. But first, we had to survive the spring, which led to the Summer from Hell! Life really is an adventure, isn't it? A roller coaster of ups and downs.

For several years, Lauren belonged to a Girl Guide Brownie group (pack), going from Sparks (SK to Grade 1) to Brownies (Grades 2 to 4). One evening in May, the girls were on a hike and Lauren fell in the ravine and landed hard on her right arm. I admit I was not terribly sympathetic to her moans. I could not figure out whether there was anything seriously wrong with her, especially since Lauren is a true creative: she's left-handed! She had not injured her dominant arm so how bad could the situation be? I told myself. I was calm and easygoing until I realized that Lauren's arm did look strange and swollen. Off to Emergency we went. The springtime hell season officially started. Lauren's arm was broken. She required surgery. She was admitted and we spent a sleepless night in a noisy hospital. I admit, it was difficult to put on a good mommy face to reassure Lauren that all would be well.

When the nurses came to take Lauren away, my stomach churned. Watching your child being taken away by a medical team is a mixed bag of feelings, dread and terror at what might happen, but also relief that your kid is getting the best possible care. Again, I feel such overwhelming waves of gratitude for being Canadian and having healthcare access. Shamus was adamant that he be the first to sign Lauren's new cast. He had come a long way since insisting his younger sibling be a boy called Andrew! Lauren's cast colours ranged from white to fluorescent pink but no matter the colour, we always had to keep her cast dry so bath time was miserable for all involved.

Lauren needing extra care and attention (affection too) added to an already stressful household. At the time, Bob was still reeling from the changes at his workplace and the imminent threat that he, like thousands of other employees and executives, would soon lose his job. His dream of a "golden handshake" had been transformed into a terrible and callous goodbye and good-luck wave. While Bob carried his burden, his daughter moped around with a cast on her arm, scratching and itching and dreading bath time. For me, managing a household and kids (and an unhappy husband), I was increasingly tired, pale, and fading fast. Only Shamus seemed to shine that spring and summer. As the temperatures hit red and humidity rolled in, Bob mostly sat around, looking glum. He had no idea what his role in life was going to look like. Each of us orbited Bob, confused and alone.

It was a happy day when Lauren's cast came off. The doctor joked, while holding a saw, that although he was still learning how to cut off casts, and not arms, he'd be careful. Lauren didn't quite burst out into tears but I knew my little girl was on the edge. What a delight that our doctor was such a jokester! Lauren's arm looked so small and white once the cast was off. There had been enough warm weather that the rest of Lauren's skin was sun-kissed with the exception of that now perfect and fully-aligned right arm.

They say bad things happen in threes: Bob losing his job, Lauren's broken arm. Two out of three. The final blow came in July. From long-time experience, I know that a clinic never calls to invite you back because your blood results are awesome. As it turned out, the blood tests showed that my creatinine levels (blood toxins) were significantly higher because my kidneys were not functioning fully. More than likely, I was warned, my kidney was generating rejection cells so a biopsy was scheduled. I wouldn't say I was happy to have a biopsy, but I sure was relieved not to have surgery. The summer was bad. Did it really need to get worse? Sadly, the universe answered, "Yes!"

I was put on bedrest for 24 hours after the biopsy. Thank goodness a very dear friend, Gloria, came and sat with me for many hours. She too was in hospital so our visits were win/win. This lovely lady was about my age. Gloria was a three-time kidney recipient. I met her when I had my first transplant while she was receiving her third. Gloria was instrumental in establishing the non-profit Canadian Transplant Association because she was so passionate about showing the world that organ recipients can work and play as functioning participants in society.

I was shocked (and so was Gloria!) that my medical team considered my kidney, transplanted 12 years earlier, was in a state of rejection. We all had been confident I'd have years of good health with zero complications or setbacks. We were wrong to believe this, especially since way back in 1983, when I received my new kidney, there were few long-term studies tracking the longevity of transplanted kidneys. My surgery was one of the few in the entire nation. Turned out my medical case was destined to be a warning (and aid) for future recipients.

With all the bad news coming down on me, I clung on even more fiercely to our summer commitment to visit Mom in Manitoba. I felt desperate to see my mother. Despite the stress of Bob losing his job, Lauren breaking her arm, and now problems with my kidney, I was committed to making our annual visit happen. Days before we were booked to fly West, the results of my biopsy came in. There were, in fact, rejection cells present in the kidney. This meant that I was to cancel our flights and our trip so I could be admitted to hospital for two weeks of IV treatment. I was not impressed. I felt fine and I wanted to spend time with my kids and my mom, not in the hospital alone. Again.

Bob and I made arrangements for Shamus and Lauren to fly to Manitoba accompanied by Mike, the kids' teenage cousin. Mike had been visiting Toronto that summer and was very much a shy country boy from rural Manitoba, who was looking forward to returning to his home province. I always liked Mike. He seemed to have a good head on his shoulders and was never wild or impulsive. Weeks earlier, our family had taken Mike to Niagara Falls for the first time. The boy's only comment was that there were "no fields" between Toronto and Niagara. You could tell he felt sorry for his city-slicker family.

When the three kids were scheduled to fly out to Winnipeg, I was given permission to accompany them to the airport. The doctors disconnected and capped my IV, so I had freedom from the pole. I escaped the hospital for a few hours. Thank goodness for small, mobile mercies. I harboured scary thoughts. My kids and their cousin would be set free inside the biggest airport in Canada and the second busiest airport in North America. I knew Shamus would take care of his little sister and I was not too worried about Mike, but kids (especially three kids) can become different people when they are on their own.

As the kids geared up for their departure gate, Bob seemed calm about the whole situation but he rarely showed emotion and certainly never in public. Me? I was a mess. I did my best to hold myself together. No kids for at least two weeks and I wasn't going to see my mom, either. The only event that awaited me was more time in the hospital. With my heart in my mouth, I bid my children goodbye, told them I loved them, and would see them in a couple of weeks. I also asked them to behave and be good to my mom. My last view of the tiny trio was them sauntering through security, Shamus confidently leading the pack with Lauren trailing behind and Mike looking astonished. I could do nothing, zero, about the situation set to unfold other than pray that God would be with them as they travelled together but alone.

Back in my hospital bed, I contemplated what my kids might be doing. I kept a close eye on the time and when I thought they would be on the plane and on their way, I breathed a little easier. Until the phone rang, and it was Shamus. How could he be calling me? He told me there had been a delay because of a thunderstorm. They were still at Pearson and had just received food vouchers as an apology for the delay, six dollars each. Shamus was clearly excited about this turn of events, especially having six bucks in his pocket to spend as he pleased. (Remember, this was 1995 and six dollars was a lot of money back then, almost $10 today.) Of course, the two boys used every single cent to stuff themselves with junk food. Lauren was unable to eat. She told me she was quite concerned about the entire situation that was unfolding. "Mommy, I am very, very worried right now," Lauren chirped into the phone.

What to do? There was nothing I could do. Again, this was the mid-90s. There was no way I could call or text my kids as they wandered the airport for hours. There was no way I could FaceTime them and reassure them that all was well. Plus, even if cellphones had existed at that time, the nurses were strict about limiting incoming and outgoing phone calls. My kids, and myself, were on their own. Shamus assured me that they'd be flying out soon and not to worry. He was 13 years old at the time, I was 39, and guess who sounded like the calm parent? Guess who sounded like a panicked child pretending to feel strong?

I immediately got on the phone to the airline to find out what was going on and to let the airline know about the kids' predicament. I was assured the children would be fine. I resisted telling the woman that was easy for her to say since it wasn't her young family running around Pearson by themselves. The agent then assured me that, in fact, the kids' flight had just taken off.

They hadn't.

I got on the phone to my mom to update her on what was going on. By this time Mike's dad had already left the farm to go to Winnipeg, a two-hour-plus drive, expecting to pick the kids up. There was no way I could contact him and tell him about the flight delay. My mom assured me over and over again that the kids would be just fine. I knew she was right, but.... There was nothing else for me to do but try to fall asleep, not something I did well in a hospital at the best of times. As you'd guess, that night was a long, restless night. I remember watching the sun rise.

I learned the next day that the kids had finally flown out of Toronto around 11 p.m., which was way past their bedtime. The grimy details emerged. The kids were giddy from fatigue and unhealthy food. Their seats were at the back of the plane so the flight attendants could keep an eye on them but that didn't stop the kids from acting silly and laughing at each other's antics. As the flight progressed, the kids were pretty much out of control and unable to stop themselves. The flight attendants suggested several times that they keep the noise down. Easier said than done when kids are overtired, unsupervised, and on some level, scared silly.

Hours later the flight touched down, finally, in Winnipeg. The kids were met by Mike's dad and his new girlfriend, who was likely a lovely woman but she was a stranger to my kids. When the girlfriend hugged Lauren, my daughter was horrified. This girlfriend was a "stranger danger!" when all Lauren wanted was to get to her Granny's and get a giant hug from someone she knew and loved. Instead, the kids suffered through a long car ride, squished together and unable to see anything but darkness. They arrived at Mom and Dudley's farm somewhere between two and three a.m. My Mom was waiting for them with all the lights on in the farmhouse. My mother, the Manitoba lighthouse, shining brightly for me and my kids during a truly hellish summer. At last, I knew my kids had found safe shelter.

Years earlier Mom commented that I expected too much of my children. She thought they were being made too responsible, burdened with making school lunches, doing laundry, and cleaning around the house. I assured her that the reason I wanted them to be independent was that I had no idea how long I would be around and able to help them. I believed strongly that my kids needed to learn how to function without me. I wanted them to cultivate the skills of creativity and initiative. Once Shamus and Lauren had been at the farm for a few days, Mom admitted that I'd raised children who were very capable and responsible. Mom was appreciative and impressed that the kids would help set the table as well as clear it after dinner. Her comment felt like something of a victory for me, even if it was in less-than-ideal circumstances. I was proud of my kids for helping, being gracious, and pulling their weight.

Meanwhile back in Toronto, I continued my IV treatment with Solumedrol (liquid Prednisone) for the full two weeks. Blood tests showed that the kidney was functioning better. Finally, I was discharged from the hospital. What a relief. My first outing was to have lunch with my dad at a restaurant on Queen Street, sitting on an outdoor patio. I always find that when I have been in hospital for some time, it is a big adjustment being out in the world again. You become so used to seeing the same walls, halls, and people that you forget how big and busy the world is. Sitting on that patio with my dad, watching all the people rushing by, felt difficult. I was grateful to be enjoying the sunshine and food with my father but as I people-watched, I couldn't help but see and feel how much poor health stole from me. I was adjusting to being back "in the world" only because I'd been excluded from it.

I gave myself a couple of days to rest at home, regain some equilibrium, and then promptly flew out toward my mom and my children. Bob and I being reunited with the kids and Mom made our visit at the farm restful and relaxing. Life felt so good, finally. Our family was reunited and we basked in Prairie summer sunshine. Even Bob, who was under such tremendous stress and disappointment, lightened up. Since we had spent time at the farm previous summers, Bob had his routine. He would help the men with chores such as harvesting crops and fixing fences. My husband stepped into such a totally different lifestyle to his usual life in the city. I was happy and relieved to see Bob enjoy his time on the farm and among the farmers. I was hopeful his good mood would last.

When we returned home from our summer vacation with Mom, life never did return to "normal." Bob and I celebrated our fifth wedding anniversary in August, but nothing felt festive or romantic. He sat in the backyard, smoking and looking depressed. I had hoped desperately that he'd remember our anniversary, but Bob didn't so our "special night" included tears of anger and hurt. Our summer hell continued unabated. You know who didn't forget our anniversary that terrible summer? Our children. Lauren and Shamus had secretly planned a celebration complete with officiant (Shamus), attendees (Lauren's stuffed animals), a flower girl (Lauren), and delicate rings (two pieces of paper inscribed with "Mom" and "Dad"). The kids' thoughtfulness was one of the sweetest things ever, which made me cry harder and longer, tears of both sadness and joy. Bob was in such a state of depression that I truly believe he was not aware of what was going on or able to appreciate the beauty around him.

I understood that Bob losing his job was a huge blow. He did receive a package which would, financially, see us through for the time being. He was offered counselling but informed me, in no uncertain terms, that he did not need help. I was welcome to talk to anybody I wanted to about my life but Bob wanted to carry his burdens alone and without support. After months of job searching, Bob started driving a truck for Canada Post. The job was right up his alley: working alone and knowing exactly where he needed to be, and at what time.

As summer shifted into fall, I realized I was unable stay in my marriage. I was grateful for the life we had together, but I knew that I could not make a relationship work all by myself. A loving connection takes two people. It was not that Bob didn't love me or value our relationship. I know he loved me. But as I watched him struggle with change and adversity, I came to realize that I could not handle the fact that he was prepared to settle for the status quo. Bob remained committed to staying in a rut. The thought of going outside his comfort zone was more than he could imagine. He had always been in control of how events in his life unfolded and he'd liked the consistency.

I, on the other hand, was anxious to try something new and different. Change for me was second nature and an aspect of life that I embraced and accepted. My resilience might have been rooted in having to move around so much as a child since I'd been a preacher's kid. Bob's upbringing had been different. He'd lived in one place until his first marriage and then only moved a time or two. Change for him was stressful and certainly not something he would choose. Bob seemed more interested in the past and how to reclaim or recreate what he believed he'd lost or had stolen from him. I saw Bob's adverse job circumstances as an opportunity for a fresh start for him, me, and our kids.

One thing I had always been interested in was owning was a B&B. While Bob was transitioning out of the insurance job and starting to look for work, we'd actually looked at a couple of places that were for sale. The majority of B&Bs were in nearby Stratford, Ontario, but Bob was adamant: as long as his mother was alive in Toronto, he would not be leaving Toronto. Period. So much for that idea. And so, the summer from hell bled into fall and winter. A new way of life for our family beckoned. There was no way I was going to live more hell. Or so I thought. I ended up staying with Bob for another six years. I bought my own house in 2001 at the ripe ole age of 45. An epic learning curve was ahead of me but at last I was living beyond the status quo and that long-ago summer from hell was finally behind me. The challenges set the course for how my life, and the lives of my children, would unfold in the years ahead. And for that, I am grateful. Each of us was growing and learning, together.

Chapter 13

Games: Me? An Athlete?

Gloria Santini and her husband were a power couple in the organ and tissue donation world. They helped found the Canadian Transplant Games Association, a charity promoting and celebrating post-transplant health. Gloria, particularly, is a hero of mine. She'd had three kidney transplants and was a passionate advocate for recipients and donors. Gloria was dedicated to removing the stigma around organ donation conversations.

In 1983 when I met Gloria, the Canadian Transplant Games Association was a small group of transplant recipients and supporters. They had a vision to spread the word about the viability of organ and tissue donation through competition at Olympic-style events. To compete in the Games, you had to have had a transplant (e.g., heart, lung, liver, kidney, pancreas, bone marrow) and be medically fit for competition. The hope was that normal, healthy, everyday people would come to watch the competitions and feel inspired to register as an organ donor. Donor family members were also invited as a way to honour their deceased loved one's gift (and still functioning organ or tissue) as well as offer support and love to the grieving family left behind.

Gloria encouraged me to become involved in the Games, either as an athlete or as part of the organizing body. My interest in either role was minimal, at best. Yet Gloria was so inspirational. She was dedicating her life to promoting the Games as a way to showcase the positive impact of "gifts of life" in Canada and around the world. As fate would have it, Canada was selected as the host country of the World Transplant Games in 1993, a solid 10 years after my first kidney transplant. The Games were to be held in Vancouver so I decided I would not only attend but also compete. The big question was, what would I compete in? I had never been athletic so there was nothing I could fall back on. Really, nothing.

I decided the "easiest" thing to do was to enter some sort of running competition. I'm not sure what made me think that running would be easy. I am not a big person and have, in fact, been described as tiny, petite, small. Not that I feel tiny, mind you. The only time I feel short is when I am standing close to a person who is really, really tall. In situations like that, I try to compensate for my height by either getting the tall person to kneel down to my level or I stand on a step or picnic table (true story). As with life, I like to look people straight in the eye as a way to remind others that although I am small, I am still mighty. Running looked more appealing than my other options. I could have competed in swimming (if I had ever been a swimmer), some sort of racquet sport like tennis, ping pong, or badminton (if I had ever picked up a racket), golf (never), or cycling (nope). You get the idea: I was not an athlete, at all. So why not just run, Forest, run. At the time, running sounded like a fabulous idea, for the most part.

Going to Vancouver was exciting. At the ripe ole' age of 37, I was staying in a university residence with approximately 100 men and women of all ages. I've never been a competitive person, yet here I was about to compete in something I was not good at, had never trained for, and had zero experience in. The one thing I had going for me? Energy and enthusiasm. Once I decided to go to the Games in Vancouver, my brother Tim, my donor, decided to go with me. Tim, bless him, had taken up running to get into shape before the kidney transplant. After our twin surgeries and his long recovery, Tim returned to running and decided to add bike-riding and swimming to his fitness training. Within a few short years after his surgery, Tim was competing in triathlons and several Iron Man competitions.

I know.

By donating his kidney to me, Tim changed his life drastically and for the better. I was proud of him and also amazed by his transformation. To say my brother took his newfound health and fitness to the extreme is putting it mildly. We both knew that having Tim attend the Games and helping out the other athletes would be fun and meaningful for him and me. My kidney donor could watch me run and cheer from the sidelines. Tim would cheer for me and must have also cheered on his transplanted kidney that was fueling and detoxifying my tiny, running body. As I expected, Tim volunteered to coach the Canadian track team. One day while we were practising various events in a nearby park, one of the heart transplant recipients fell to the ground. Since this was long before cell phones, I ran as I have never run before in search of a phone to call 911. I ran to the nearest home and banged on their door, the adrenaline taking over. We learned later that heart transplant recipients have no nerve connections and therefore feel no pain. The young man who'd experienced the heart incident was okay, but he wouldn't be running or competing anytime soon. The man's misfortune hit close to home. Our older brother David had died from a heart attack at 37 (the age I was while competing in Vancouver). David had dropped dead while running a race. And now here I was, semi-sickly and definitely small, about to hear the trigger pulled and run, Melody, run. Life sure is as precious as it is fragile.

To this day I wonder why I chose to run track. I believe I now know my answer. I wanted to honour my brothers, David and Tim. One brother was dead and missed dearly. My other brother had driven half-way across the country to coach me and cheer from the sidelines. Wouldn't it be nice to imagine that David was "up there" cheering me on too?

I realized soon after arriving at the Games that the other recipients were "my people." I felt so at home. There was no need to try to fit in since I immediately felt like I belonged, which was both a surprising and wonderful feeling. When transplant recipients meet, the conversation goes something like this, "What are you?" or "What have you had?" Most people ask what your astrological sign is, what you do for a living, or start some other boring chitchat inquiry. Transplant people? No topic is too personal. Take, for example, some of our favourite opening lines when we meet new transplant people: What organ have you received? What illness changed your life? How'd you strike back against illness? With a new heart, liver, kidney, etc.? We all had similar experiences, but none of our healthcare journeys was the same.

A lot of the people competing at the Games had once been healthy and then suddenly were deathly ill. As Tim and I listened to people's stories, it was impossible not to appreciate and be in awe of just how miraculous organ donation is. People who were at death's door were returned, usually through the generosity and kindness of a stranger, to being healthy and strong because of a "gift of life." One of my favourite stories was from a young woman who'd been a competitive swimmer in high school. She developed liver disease, needed a liver transplant, received the gift, and now? The woman returned to swimming within months and has gone to win multiple Games medals for her competitive swimming. And look at me, if we must. (And I know, we've been looking at me throughout this memoir.) Here I was, Melody Klassen, sickly her whole life yet still running around like an athlete and surrounded by people just like me. In the transplant crowd, I was similar not special. Fitting in and not being an anomaly was such a blessing and relief.

Despite having the best coach and cheerleader (Tim), I was still me. Moments before the race, I tripped and fell. Over what? Who knows. I tend to be clumsy. My scrape-up was just me being me. When it was time for my event, the 100-metre, I stood at the start line taking deep breaths. Not only was I going to run, I was going to sprint as fast as I could. If I hadn't been so nervous, I would have laughed out loud at the ridiculousness! Before I knew it and long before I was ready, the starter pistol blasted off. My fellow competitors and I were literally off to the races. I was proud that I finished the race. As expected, I didn't win the race but you know what? I didn't place last, which was such an accomplishment. Almost as good? Finishing the race and looking over and seeing my big brother Tim clapping and cheering for me. Thank you, Tim, for supporting me. Thank you, Gloria, for building something so beautiful for people like us.

Forever Grateful

A number of years after our Vancouver World Games, Gloria told me she had cancer. As was her style, my dear friend fought with all she had. There were lots of people praying for her recovery. Sadly, Gloria's fight was over. Her race had come to a close before the new millennium. It's always hard when one of your friends, a piece of your social circle, dies. Death brings home, as it always does irrespective of the circumstances, just how fragile life is. For people like me and Gloria, life is especially tender since we're well-aware we are living on borrowed time. We are alive because of a gift, the gift of organ donation. I was fortunate to play my harp at Gloria's funeral. What an honour to play at my friend's send-off but how hard knowing we'd never see her smile or hear her laughter ever again. The majority of the funeral attendees went home carrying deep sorrow but also a deep and renewed commitment to promoting organ and tissue donation. Gloria had been so dedicated and passionate and now we, her friends and family, would carry that torch and shine light on the importance of gifting people with "gifts of life." As some of us like to joke, you can't take your organs with you. Give them away and save lives.

There had been so much fun in Vancouver. Plenty of laughter and tears, late nights, karaoke catastrophes, friendly competition, and to-be-lifelong camaraderie. I admit, it was a bit of a letdown heading home to Toronto. I had missed my family, but I had been free of responsibility in Vancouver, a welcome relief and respite for a mother of a young and rambunctious family. Shamus was 11, Lauren was five, and my marriage to Bob continued to toil and trouble. Coming home with so much joy to share made my mother's absence even more overwhelming. There were plenty of phone calls to Manitoba but so many times I hung up the phone and wished desperately that Mom lived with us or at least in the same city.

I decided the best way to keep my positive mindset was to continue my involvement with the Games. I was elected to the National Board for the Canadian Transplant Association (the Games rebranded so the charity was more inclusive to less able-bodied folks) as recording secretary. My volunteer role was a fun way to stay involved, give back, see my new friends, and stay current about research and new initiatives happening in the transplant world. I loved the CTA so it came to no one's surprise when I aligned my family more deeply with one of my greatest passions.

In 2000 the first-ever Canadian Transplant Games were held in Sherbrooke, Québec. Approximately 80 transplant recipients competed with an impressive number of friends and family in attendance and competing too! We were showing the world (or at least people in Québec) that organ donation and transplantation change lives and build community. For me, the most memorable event at the Games was during the relay race. Our family had put together a team: Shamus, Lauren, Tim, and me. When it was my turn to run, I literally got off on the wrong foot and popped my hamstring. When I fell, Tim bolted over, patted me on the shoulder, grabbed the baton, and carried on. We did reasonably well, considering. There's sure nothing wrong with a shiny silver medal shared among family.

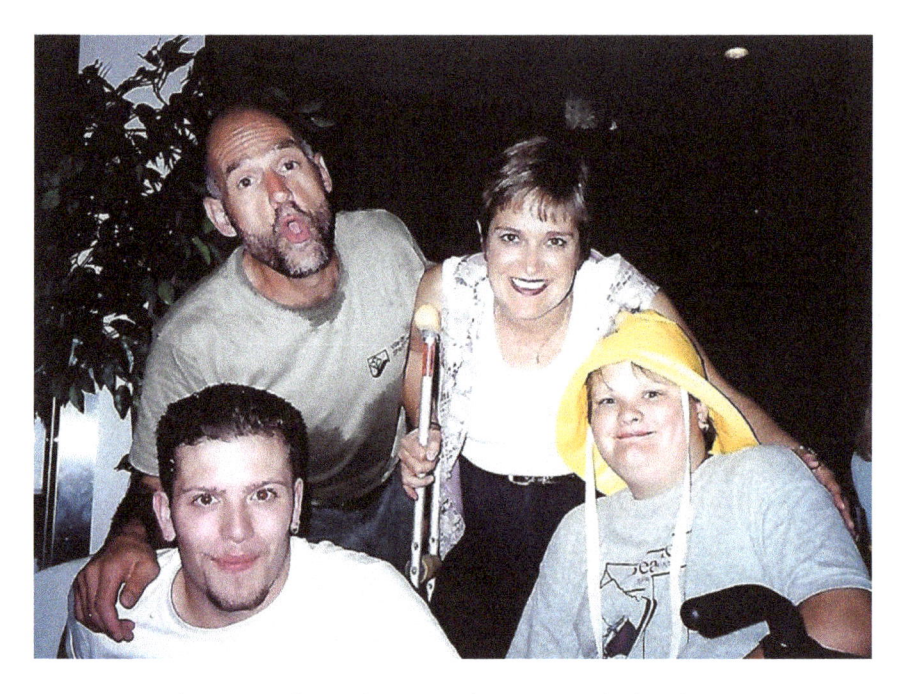

At the inaugural Canadian Transplant Games, Sherbrooke, 2000
(L to R) Tim, Me, Shamus, Lauren

In 2005 London, Ontario, hosted our World Games at Western University. Over 1500 participants from 46 countries attended, accompanied by family, friends, and curious spectators. The most revered guests were donor family members (i.e., their loved one had died and given gifts of life) and living donors (e.g., kidney and liver donors). The sporting events were well organized and efficiently run. And the fun after-hours social events were exceptional, whether a cowboy/cowgirl dinner where we were encouraged to dress up and say "yeehaw" a lot, or an impressive pub crawl through the city. Unlike most of the athletes (I was a lawn bowler), my kids attended the Games and proved themselves to be boisterous and dedicated cheerleaders. "Good shot, Mom! Way to go!" was a constant cheer as I competed against my (hungover) fellow athletes. As fate would have it, the Games' famous pub crawl had been the night before. My winning edge, although I didn't win, was that I am not a big drinker so I enjoyed bowling on the green but didn't look green! I was thrilled and proud to have Shamus and Lauren with me that trip. A family that plays together, stays together.

Gloria's legacy took centre stage in our family as the years unfolded. In 2006 Lauren and I attended the Canadian Games in Edmonton. En route to being spectators, we toured around Calgary. What a delight to revisit my old stomping grounds after so many decades away. It was fun taking my 18-year-old daughter down Memory Lane. She was just a bit younger than I had been when 23-year-old me made the move across the country, from Toronto to Calgary, to start a new life. Lauren and I also visited Wetaskiwin, a tiny town we'd lived in before Mom and Dad moved me and my brothers to Toronto. (What Lauren and I didn't know then was that we were destined to revisit Memory Lane again, in 2012, at the Calgary Games; a visit when I could show her my mountains: Banff and Lake Louise. I refrained from sharing my tales of mischief, mountains, and men!)

The final event of the Edmonton Games was a gala dinner and a very Alberta-style dish was served: buffalo. My vegetarian daughter was aghast and then even more so when her meat was replaced by mushrooms, a vegetable (fungi, actually!) we both detest. I must confess, I laughed. Lauren remained unimpressed but we both maintain to this day that our Alberta trip was special and one of a kind.

Although I'd hurt myself in Florida and missed competing in the 2008 Windsor Games, I was still awarded a gold medal from the safety of the sidelines! A lovely Games competitor, and fellow kidney recipient, gifted me their gold. I'd always made the joke that I'd win a gold in socializing, and in a way, I did. Yet despite how chatty I am, I was gobsmacked and overcome with emotion when I was crowned in gold. The joy the Games brought to my life never ceased to amaze me. For example, Québec City hosted the 2010 Games where I competed in 10-pin bowling and pétanque (a type of lawn bowling). Not once did I knock down a single pin in bowling.

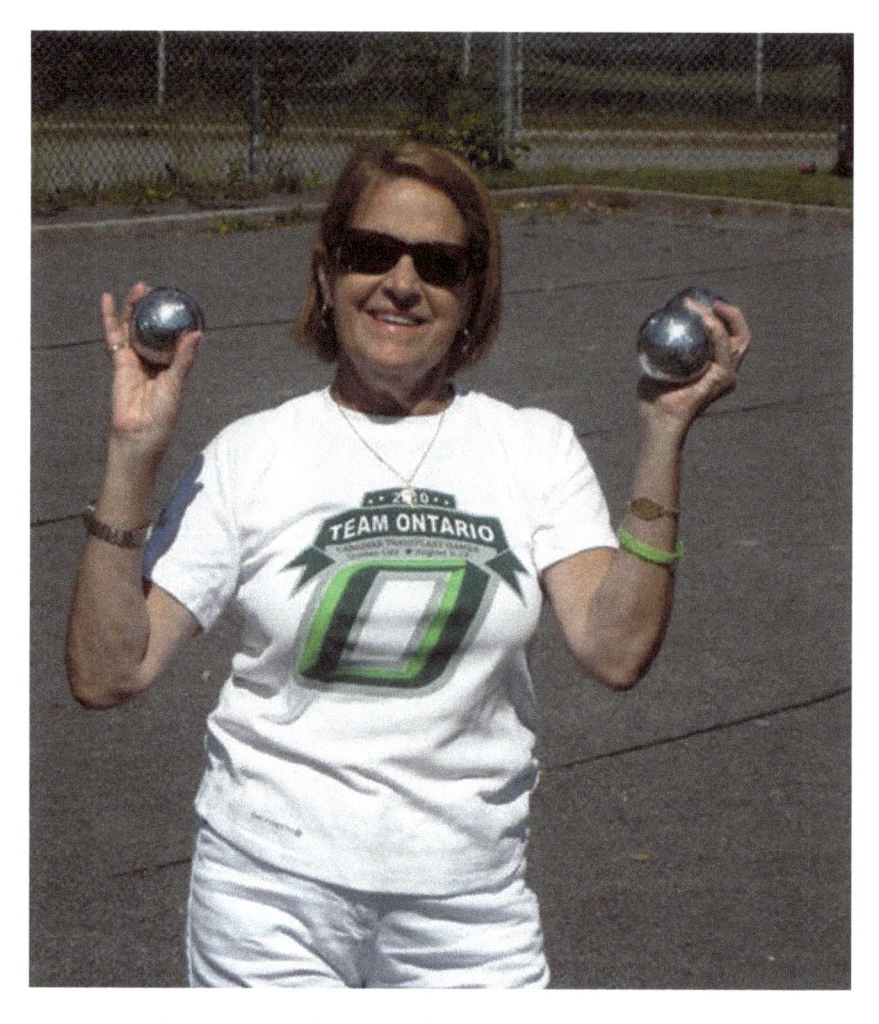

Me at the Canadian Transplant Games, Quebec City, 2010
Showing off my Petanque skills

How funny is that? A French love theme developed throughout 2010. I travelled to Paris and southern France, another opportunity to revisit a special time in my youth. Shamus and April were married that same year. Again, I am blessed.

As much as I attribute my love of the Canadian Transplant Association and the Games to my friend Gloria, I also always think of my brother Tim. Right from the beginning of my "athletic career," Tim was by my side, cheering me on. I wonder what it was like for him, watching me run around and thrive while knowing his kidney was inside of me, making me happy and healthy? In the late 90s, the CTA decided to start up a transplant dragon boat team. One of our members was a world-class dragon boater and it was her inspiration, guidance, and perseverance that birthed Team Transplant. Every time we were in a dragon boat race, paddling out to the starting line, I felt nervous and nauseated. I was worried I would let the rest of my team down. Not that it all depended on me, of course, since there were 20 of us in the boat and most of my teammates were bigger and stronger than I. Dragon boat racing was great fun and Tim, again cheering on little sister, was our dedicated steers person.

That first year at the Dragon Boat Festival Tim and I were interviewed by the Toronto Star newspaper. "Brother and sister are in the same boat" read the headline. I absolutely lovedseeing Tim recognized nationally for his gift of (kidney) life to me. We were having fun, raising awareness, and helping others. What made our training and competing even more challenging was that the dragon boat circuit was not "donor recipient only." Our team was the minority since everyone else was "normal" (organ and tissue donor-free) so we took great delight in living in the moment and letting the world know we were alive, healthy, and present.

Our team's ultimate goal, beyond winning races, was to inspire Canadians to register as organ donors. Whether I played my harp at ceremonies honouring lost loved ones or having one-on-one conversations with strangers, I quickly realized organ donation is a lightning rod for a lot of people. I remember one year I was approached by a man at the Dragon Boat Festival. He asked me who my team was and why we were considered so special and different from the other teams.

I told him that my teammates and I had all received life-saving organ transplants. We chatted for a few minutes before I asked him if he was a registered donor. He looked horrified and made it clear that he was not and never would be. I asked him if one of his loved ones ever needed a transplant, what would he do? He assured me that if anyone in his family needed a transplant, they would get one, absolutely.

Interesting, isn't it?

For some people it's more than okay to need and receive a transplant, in fact most people feel entitled to receive life-saving organs and tissues. But it's borderline disdainful and crass to register for donation and offer that same gift to others upon your death. That ridiculous man from so many years ago still makes me shake my head. Sadly, people like that are legion around the world. But don't worry, I have a solution. Canada would benefit from following Spain's lead, which has enacted "presumed consent" into law. In other words, when you die in Spain, medical professionals presume you've consented to donate any and all viable organs and/or tissues. If a citizen wishes not to be a donor, they must have completed paperwork, etc., clearly showing their medical wishes. As of writing these pages, Canada still has an archaic system that allows grieving, traumatized family members to override their deceased loved one's donation wishes!

I've heard terrible stories over the years of Canadian families declaring war on one another because they can't agree on what the deceased wanted done with their organs and tissues. And the real rub? As a Canadian, if you're not clear about your desire to offer a gift of life, people die. I know that sounds dramatic but the stakes are that high, life and death. If you already haven't agreed to be a donor, you can easily register at www.beadonor.ca. Contributing to your legacy in this way takes less than five minutes. All you need is your health card, a splash of courage and bravery, and the willingness to follow-up with your family and tell them what you've done and what you want done (and your wishes honoured) upon your transition from life to afterlife. Your beautiful body may help save up to 75 lives because of your organ and/or tissue donation. If this is your decision, bless you.

I think the biggest hurdle for most people when thinking about organ donation is looking at the conundrum of life: we are born, we live, and we die. When we die (spoiler alert: not "if"), we leave a footprint, a legacy. What better way than to live this life and know you've saved lives? Every moment I am alive, whether running relay, striking out at lawn bowling, or dragon-boat racing, I am thankful for the gift of my kidneys. My love for this precious gift and this fragile life is everlasting. There is joy in being able to help others, now and in the afterlife. Organ donation is truly the ultimate gift of life.

Chapter 14

Unbelievable: Grandkids

I love this Irish saying, "Children are the rainbow of life, grandchildren are the pot of gold."

I must admit that I had never given any thought to having grandchildren. My parents had been blessed with grandchildren and openly addressed the grandkids as "our dreams come true." My four brothers and I had all done our part to maintain the world's population, with a total of nine children among us.

Having children was such an amazing and unexpected experience that it never really occurred to me that someday I might also become a grandparent. What I wanted above all else for my kids? That they be happy and healthy. And make wise life choices about how they spend their time and with whom. Shamus and I had always had a close and special relationship. I knew that someday he would choose a life partner. My concern was: who would that someone be? While Shamus was studying Drama at Queen's University, he met a lovely young woman. They were cheerleading partners (true story) and got to know each other while doing lifts and jumps. At the time of their courtship, April was studying Science at Queen's. After completing her Bachelor of Education, April started teaching.

My daughter-in-law is a wonderful human being and fits in well with our tight-knit family. Lauren and I knew April was a keeper the first time we met her. It was Christmas and we were doing a jigsaw puzzle when she walked into the room on Shamus' arm. She came over and dove right in, loving puzzles as much as we did!

April and Shamus chose to live together for a couple of years. The fact that Shamus's dad and I had divorced made Shamus anxious about jumping into marriage. Yet after they had been living together for just over six months, Shamus confided that he could not imagine living his life without April. He was going to propose at Christmas. If Shamus was that sure, I was with him and smiled broadly and happily as he told me his plans. After the annual Christmas Eve celebration at April's parents' house, once they were alone in their apartment, Shamus proposed. The young couple decided they would have a long engagement, over a year and a half, so there would be lots of time to plan the perfect wedding.

Their August 2010 nuptials was the best party! Every detail had been taken care of and carefully shared with guests. The celebration was formal but also low-key and lots of fun. There were about 150 people in attendance, a perfect number, considering April is from a big family and Shamus has us and his dad. The ceremony and reception were held at the Arcadian Court in downtown Toronto. Once the papers were signed and "Mr. and Mrs. Fynes" officially introduced, hors d'oeuvres were served. A delicious dinner and joyful dancing followed. The speeches were short and to the point. Shamus did a wonderful job introducing his family, not an easy task.

Shamus and I danced to "What a Wonderful World," a special favourite of my dad's. We were both in tears, wishing Dad was there with us. Adrian (Shamus's dad) and I had been divorced for almost 25 years and, of course, both of us were at the wedding. I must admit there were some awkward moments. He and his partner chose to sit apart from me during the ceremony and there are no pictures with Adrian, me, Shamus, and April. I am glad that we were both able to be there and celebrate the happiness of our son, even if we were unable to celebrate together.

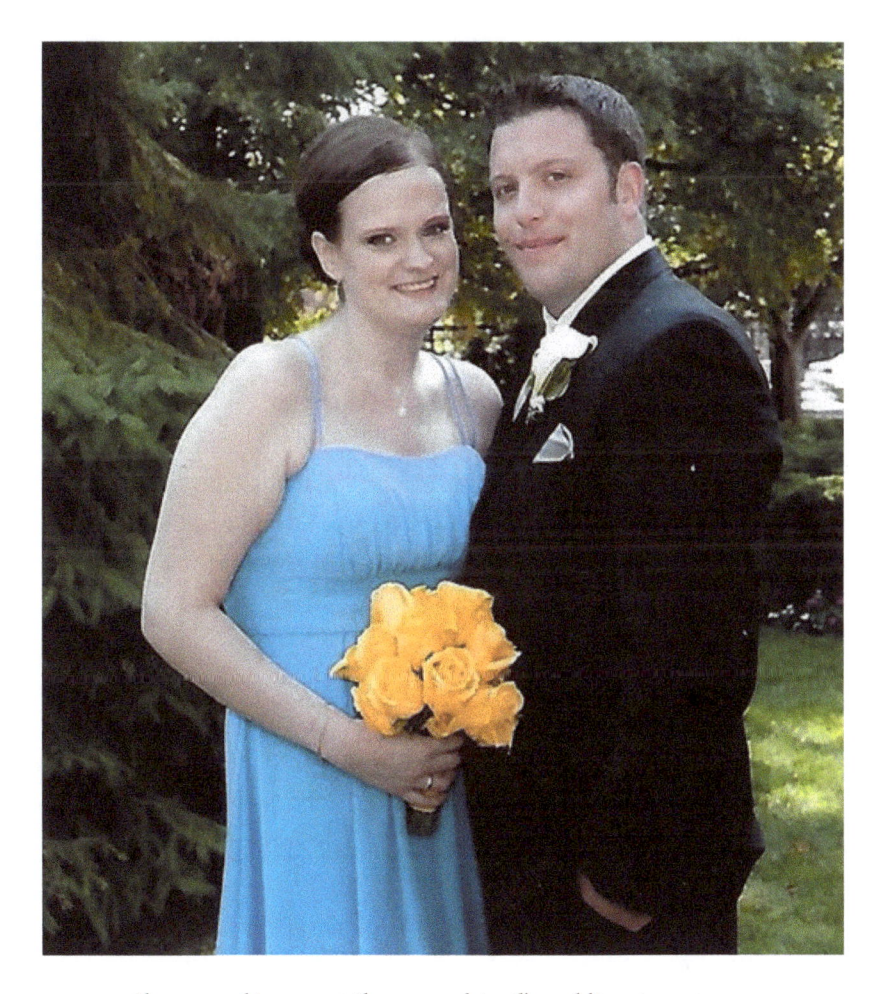

Shamus and Lauren at Shamus and April's wedding, August 2010

From the onset, Shamus and April were clear on how they wanted things to go in their lives: get married, buy a house, and have children. Exactly eight years after my second kidney transplant, June 12th, 2011, Lauren and I were invited for dinner at Shamus and April's. When we arrived, Shamus handed us each an envelope. Strange. What was going on? Tentatively I opened mine and pulled out a single sheet of paper, which read "Grandma Got Run Over by a Reindeer," one of our family's favourite Christmas songs. Click. I was going to be a grandma. My face lit up and I did a happy dance right there in their kitchen. I was going to be a grandma.

Meanwhile, Lauren had opened her envelope and inside she found the song lyrics to "The Ants go Marching In." Lauren was going to be an aunt! Such a unique way to share and spread wonderful news. Lauren and I were famous, possibly notorious, for breaking into song spontaneously. The tradition was just something we did, whether we were alone at home or attending Transplant Games events! Shamus and April taking the time to match song titles to their baby news felt extra special and super personal. I can't resist: their delivery was melodious and pitch perfect.

How do I explain what it feels like to begin a day with the intention of celebrating my eighth transplant anniversary and ending the day with the news I was going to be a granny? As a day to celebrate and rejoice. A day to deeply remember and honour the fact that each day of life is a gift. I wish there were another word for "gratitude" that could fully express my joy, then and now. "Carpe diem," seize the day, is important advice for all of us, especially those blessed with a transplant that's keeping them alive and healthy.

Amazement, happiness, joy, love. These are just some of the feelings that bubbled inside me as I considered life as a granny. We were going to have another member in our family. There was much hugging and actual jumping for joy, the night of the announcement and for many months afterwards. The excitement I felt while I'd been pregnant with Shamus and Lauren had never been matched until that baby announcement in 2011. Finding out a grandchild was coming into our lives opened up new dimensions of joy and trust in the miracle of life, love, and family.

April told me that the expected delivery date of "our" baby was set for February 11th, Shamus's birthday. As exciting as it would have been for the baby to arrive on their Daddy's birthday, I really hoped that the baby wouldn't. Everyone deserves to have their own special day, a day for Shamus to be celebrated with a cake just for him. Only time would tell if the baby made his or her appearance before, during or after new Daddy's birthday.

April's pregnancy went smoothly. The to-be parents moved into their first home that summer. Christmas came and went, and the due date grew ever closer. So did our family's excitement. As the New Year was rung in, Shamus and April knew a baby girl was destined to take centre stage soon. My son's birthday arrived, Shamus's 30th, and the baby decided not to overshadow her Daddy's big day. "Our" baby girl decided to give her father his due, so Shamus's birthday remained his own. But a week later, the newest member of our family let us all know it was time to prepare for her arrival. Shamus called us early in the morning and announced they were en route to the hospital. In the excitement of that phone call, I forgot to ask how they were all doing. Was April in a lot of pain? Was Shamus okay to drive to the hospital? Was there any sense of timing? Did Lauren and I need to hurry or could we take our time getting across town to the hospital? Lauren was anxious to get to the hospital as soon as humanly possible. She had no intention of missing the birth of her niece! This ant/aunt was marching right in!

It was a long day for everyone, hanging out at the hospital. We were all there: Shamus, Lauren, me, April's parents. (Shamus's dad and his long-time partner were snowbirds in Florida that winter.) Finally, she arrived. At 3:13 p.m. on February 18th, 2012, Emma Grace was born. The wait was over. Emma was among us, named after Shamus's dearly loved and departed friend. We were all allowed into the birthing suite as soon as April was ready to receive visitors. Each of us took a turn holding Emma, just minutes after she was born. Emma was, of course, beautiful with a full head of dark hair and the right number of fingers and toes. Such happiness for all of us.

We were forever changed. There was a baby in our midst, the first grandchild on both sides. Emma was a much-loved baby immediately and now I was forever a granny. Even after several years, it is still hard to grasp that not only do I have two children, but I also am blessed with little people who call me "Granny," enjoy spending time with me, and get excited when I walk into the room (and notice when I leave). I have always been amazed by the miracle of birth and how we grow, but when life is changing so drastically and beautifully within your own family, life is even more fascinating. My love of babies has always filled me with deep, loving emotion. Every time I saw Baby Emma in those first few months, she had grown and changed. Her brown expressive eyes changed and twinkled with each passing week. Before too long, she was no longer a newborn.

The near-constant question on my and Lauren's minds: how long before we could host Emma for a sleepover and take her places? We lived on the other side of the city from Shamus and April, so it was time-consuming to reach Emma's house. Dropping in for a quick baby snuggle was challenging and often impossible. Yet there were some evenings when I'd decide I just absolutely needed to see my granddaughter, and her parents too, of course. After dinner I would sometimes jump in the car and drive across town like the devil himself was after me. My love for Emma fueled the drive. My impulse visits were always worth it. Just to hold Emma, maybe even change a diaper, and whisper how much I loved her filled me with such grace and gratitude. I simply had not known how much love my heart could hold and share until I met Emma.

I was constantly amazed by how she grew and changed between visits. With each passing month, the distance between our two houses seemed further and further away. Commuting to see Emma was especially difficult for full-time working Lauren, who very much wanted to be a full-time "Ant Who Marched In." Before we could believe it, Emma was an active toddler. I loved being with her and just admiring the way Emma grew and learned. She was truly a sponge. As a parent, watching your own children is different from watching your grandchildren. When I was with Emma, I didn't have a million things I needed or wanted to do. I savoured just being with Emma, nothing else, no one else. That little girl had my undivided, loving attention.

As Emma's motor skills developed, we read stories and did puzzles. Like her mother, grandmother, and aunt, Emma loved puzzling, then and now. A year-and-a-half later, as we toasted Canada Day in Shamus and April's backyard, Shamus very quietly announced that April was pregnant again. It was early in her pregnancy and they were surprised that conception had happened so quickly. Shamus shared the news so quietly, in fact, that at first I did not really register what he was saying. Then, I realized that April had foregone the traditional Canada Day champagne. More joy, excitement, and happiness to come. We were all so thrilled that Emma was going to be a big sister.

There is a strange phenomenon in my family. Each of my nieces and nephews who've had more than one child always produce a matching brother or sister. So, for example, if your first child is a son, the next baby you have will be a little boy. If your first is a daughter, get ready for another baby girl. My oldest niece has two girls, my next niece has two boys, and so on. An interesting occurrence. Maybe fodder for a PhD thesis? The big question in our family? Was Emma predestined to have a baby sister? I've never been much of a gambler but I was convinced that Shamus and April were going to break the boy-boy, girl-girl pattern and produce a son for themselves, a grandson for me. The couple might have been swayed by my amateur fortune telling. Shamus and April debated potential boys' names for quite some time until they had tangible ultrasound-proof that they were having a girl. Our mysterious and magical family-birthing pattern continues!

Arrangements had been made for Lauren to go and stay with Emma once her future baby sister was set to make her appearance. Despite being in her mid-twenties and busy, Lauren absolutely loved spending time with her two-year-old niece, her "munchkin." They had a lovely rapport and relationship so I was always delighted to admire Lauren and Emma when they were together. It was easy, and wonderful, to imagine how Lauren will one day interact with her own children, whenever that special time comes.

Mid-March in Toronto delivers rain or snow (or both!). On March 12th, the city was blanketed in gorgeous snow, which made for an adventurous drive toward April, who was having mild but regular contractions. After a short visit and leaving Lauren behind with Emma and her parents, I headed back home not knowing when the actual delivery would happen. Later that night, around midnight, Shamus called and informed me they were heading to the hospital. I figured I had a little bit of time before my grand baby showed up, so I rolled over and expected to snuggle back to sleep for a few more hours. But just as I fell asleep, I started having pangs of pain in my lower left abdomen, which usually signified diverticulitis, an intestinal infection. I ignored my body's warning bells and showed up at the hospital around 2:30 a.m. with less than an hour to spare before Lily Kathryn entered this world with a cry and probably a giggle too. March 13th, 2014, was another magical day in my life.

Again, there was such excitement, joy, and happiness for all of us. We were blessed with the opportunity to hold Lily so soon after her arrival, a true moment in time for me and our entire family. An overwhelming feeling of "Does life get any better?" was only tempered by the growing flare-up in my abdomen. Full-blown diverticulitis had arrived. My intestines felt as if they were on fire and being stabbed at the same time. Physical pain and poor health once again threatened to overshadow my happiness. But no level of suffering could diminish my joy and love as I met and celebrated the arrival of newborn Lily. For that joy-infused focus, I am grateful.

Chapter 15

Grand Parenthood: What Fun

Pain in the lower left quadrant of my abdomen. Indication of diverticulitis. Give my pain a number out of 10? I'd say eight or nine. I was able to make it through the night and hold myself together until after Lily was born. But shortly after our loving introduction, I found a hospital bench and promptly stretched out, hoping that by lying still, I could get the pain to go away. It didn't. Instead, the pain grew and grew some more. With diverticulitis, the lower-left abdomen starts cramping then escalates quickly, as if a knife is being plunged into your gut and twisted, again and again.

When I know that I am in need of an Emergency Department, I tend to make my way to St. Michael's since they have all my records. (Lily was not born at my "favourite" hospital, which was fine with me. I loved not visiting St. Mike's, especially on happy occasions!) With the help of a dear friend, I was in the Emergency Dept at St. Mike's by mid-morning the day that Lily was born. The commute was worth it since the doctors and nurses at St. Mike's always keep my compromised immune system in mind when offering treatment. Happily, I was away from the baby festivities for only a few hours, since I was able to convince the doctor to give me antibiotics and let me go. Freedom!

My joy at being present at the birth of my second granddaughter was beyond belief. I know that my crazy body has its issues, and there are times when I feel betrayed by my poor health, but this time I held my body and mind together. I was able to hold command over the pain and not share with Shamus and April what was happening with me. To this day I am grateful that nothing overshadowed or splintered their happiness as they welcomed Lily into their family.

I knew from previous experience with diverticulitis that once the doctors made a definitive diagnosis (done) and began a treatment of antibiotics (done), it was only a matter of a day or two before the pain subsided. Years before when I encountered the screaming "fun" that is diverticulitis, I had two options: stay in hospital for another couple of days or go to a comedy show with Lauren. Guess which decision I made? Exactly. I figured that laughter would be a great healer and I suppose my doctors did too. Even with another round of diverticulitis showing up, I was still so grateful for the life I was living. Now not only do I have two children, I am blessed with two grandchildren. There are few words to describe the feelings that swell up inside me when I remember the girls being welcomed into this world. Imagine that I once had been a young woman, a teenager really, being told I'd never have a family of my own. And now? I am so blessed by a blossoming family tree with deep, strong roots.

I chose to be called "Granny" because my mom had been "Granny" (more specifically, "Granny K"). Mom had died a year before Emma was born so she never had the delight of meeting her great grandchildren. She did not have the pleasure of meeting the "girlies" and loving them as I do. Every time I hear the girls call me "Granny," which is often, I feel like on some level I am honouring my mother and their great-grandmother, Granny and Granny K. I love that sad but strong ode to the love from the past, which warms us and holds us tight today.

Emma and Lily certainly "know" my parents through pictures. They know that they were Granny's mom and dad. My parents are known as Great Papa Wesley and Great Granny Ina. Death is a challenging concept to discuss with children, especially highly intelligent and intuitive children like my girlies. I have been asked more than once the following:

Forever Grateful

When Great Granny Ina is back from being dead, can we see her? Can we call your mommy on the phone today, Granny? If only, Emma and Lily. I really wish Granny could call her Mommy and her Daddy too. And the phone calls to heaven wouldn't stop there, would they? I wish my girlies could have met my brother David and known Jay.

When I was growing up, we did not live close to my grandparents. We moved to Ontario when I was three and my two grandmothers lived in Manitoba and Saskatchewan. We were lucky if we saw either of them once a year. I knew no grandfathers. My paternal grandfather died when my dad was 16 and my mom's dad died when I was only three. I feel like I missed out on a lot by not knowing my grandfathers and I wish I'd had a chance to be more influenced (and spoiled?) by my grandmothers. I was always grateful that my kids had such a deep and involved relationship with my parents, their grandparents. My dad spent a lot of time with Shamus and Lauren just hanging out, playing games (Dad taught them how to play Mancala), reading, and talking. Both Shamus and Lauren have fond memories of their time with their beloved Papa.

Having grandparents adds a layer of history to our lives and gives children a different perspective on the world. Kids are pretty much guaranteed unconditional love from grandparents, who simply don't have the stress and burden of parenting. Being a grandparent is fun and flexible without any of the hustle and bustle of early mornings, homework duties, teenage moods, or (gasp!) dating.

Considering the impact of my parents on my kids' lives, it's no wonder I was committed to staying present in my grandchildren's lives. I had excellent role models.

Once Lily was born, Lauren and I decided we'd sell our house in the east end and buy a condo in the west end of Toronto so we could be closer to Shamus's family of precious girls. One of the funny things about Toronto is that people who live in the east end are usually lifelong East Enders, sometimes extending back several generations. The same tradition unfolds in the west end. There was much incredulity from my east end friends that we were leaving and moving across the city. But most of our social circle had met Emma and knew that Lily was en route. My friends knew the competition was stiff! I enjoyed the teasing since it was good-natured and celebratory. I was moving away but I knew I'd take my friends with me, at least inside my heart. All those passionate East Enders knew there was a lot of beauty and love waiting for me and Lauren in the west end.

It's been almost a decade since Lauren and I moved and the west end is absolutely where I belong. I love where I live. I see the girls as often as I can. Lauren and I are available to help with the girls at a moment's notice because we live only minutes away. If one of my granddaughters is sick, we can help out immediately. If one of them needs to be picked up at school, we're waiting at the curb. When the girls are at home and their parents are working, Lauren and I are at the door, ready to roll for the day, which we've nicknamed "Camp Grauntie" days.

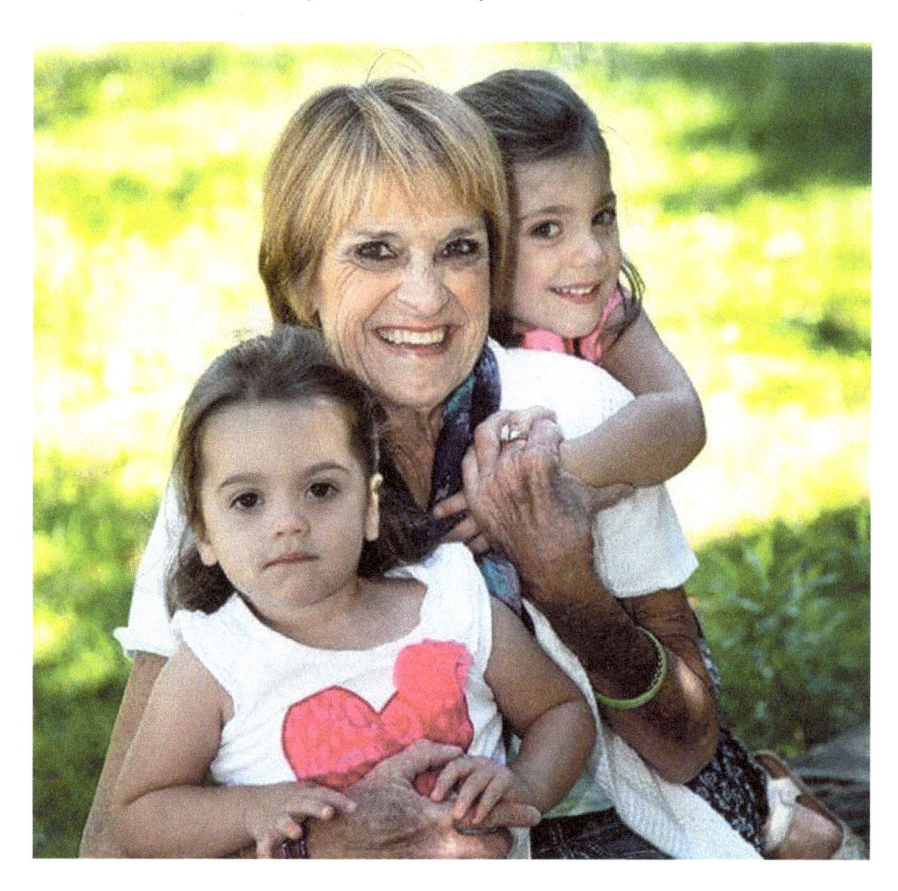

Emma (4), Lily (2) and I, summer 2016

The girls love doing crafts and Lauren does her best to create a craft studio equipped with crafty ideas that must entertain two nieces all day. Whether it's making a mason-jar snow globe or braiding bracelets, my girlies always have a craft to enjoy, make, and present to their parents by day's end. (Shamus and Lauren were deprived of crafts growing up. I apologize for nothing. I have an aversion to getting my hands dirty or sticky.) Craft making is usually followed by cookie making, all of us squeezed into the kitchen. Baking creations range from shortbread for Christmas to heart-shaped Jam Jams for Valentine's Day. Baking with my three girls activates such nostalgia in me. I absolutely adored baking with my mom both as a child and as a grown-up.

Another bonus about living close to Emma and Lily is that Lauren teaches her nieces piano and singing. My daughter is such a good teacher and relates so well to children of all ages, especially her two favourite students! Another favourite pastime is hosting our girlies for sleepovers. I make a point of telling stories that teach the girls about our family history as well as showing them what their dad was like when he was a kid. During sleepovers, Lauren and I become girls ourselves. Whether we're doing "Build-a-Bear" marathon sessions, riding bikes, visiting the park, drawing pictures, reading to one another, or throwing the ball around, our time together passes quickly and joyfully. The four of us will venture out to PetSmart for hours to admire everything that lives and breathes inside the store: fish, birds, guinea pigs, hamsters, kittens, and puppies. Poor creatures stuck at "pet daycare" are also admired and coveted: "No, girls. We cannot take that dog home. That is someone else's pet not yours."

Emma is very much like her dad in looks as well as temperament. Shamus was always an entertainer and Emma is clearly following and dancing in his footsteps. She always has a joke to share or a song to sing. With Emma directing, the two girls regularly stage some sort of recital that involves dancing, singing, and a few jokes. They love to perform for whomever is sitting on the couch, and happily for me and Lauren, we are the girls' biggest fans and most devoted audience members!

Lily, the youngest, has a great sense of humour. At the time of this writing, Lily is seven, big sister Emma is nine. Lily is a dear soul, possibly an old soul. She and her ant/auntie Lauren have a special bond. We call

Lauren the "Lily Whisperer" because she's always been able to calm Lily when she is upset. It's so lovely seeing my daughter and youngest granddaughter together. Whenever the four of us go out for a walk, Lily confidently slips her hand into Lauren's, looks up, and grins.

Emma and Lily are quite different. Recently the two girls decided they'd like to attend church with me. When it was time for the children to go downstairs to attend their (fun) Sunday School, Emma was out of the pew immediately, ready to go. Lily, on the other hand, snuggled up closer to me and whispered she was staying right where she was, with Granny. While Emma is confident when it comes to new situations and people, Lily takes her time getting comfortable. Eventually Lily did join Emma downstairs but not a second before she was ready and willing. Watch out, world! My girlies are brave, tender hearts; small and mighty like their Granny and the women before them.

Being a grandparent is an important role I take seriously. I can offer Emma and Lily love, patience, and acceptance without the stress Mom and Dad face. As the girls get older, there are more things we'll do together. For example, I look forward to taking them to musical concerts and theatrical performances. We can take advantage of outdoor fun and venture further from home. Right now the girls love riding their bikes while Granny walks behind. I'm given such a lift in mind, body, and spirit when I watch the girls take swimming lessons, play baseball, and chase after soccer balls. The girls don't skate as much as bolt around the rink, fast as lightning and just as bright and sparkling. Quiet time together includes some of my favourite long-time hobbies: reading aloud, doing puzzles, playing boardgames. My granddaughters are smart, funny, intelligent, precocious, and delightful. They make me laugh, they fill my life with joy and love.

And they positively and happily exhaust me. There is a good reason why women over 55 do not have children. We run out of energy long before children do!

Emma and Lily are growing and developing as human beings so quickly. To think that I might miss even part of their lives is unthinkable. I always want them to know I love them unconditionally and forever. A big part of my life is dedicated to showing the girls that they can call me anytime and ask me anything. I want my girlies to know in the marrow of their bones that Granny will always be there for them, love them, and cherish them. I am filled with such gratitude to be part of their lovely lives.

I never know what the girls will say or do. As they grow older, will the sisters be friends or foes as they chase a soccer ball or play in the tub? It's fun watching the sisterly dynamics and dynamite! What remains the same no matter what? Emma and Lily will always be sisters. They'll always be known, deeply and lovingly, by a sibling who loves them. As sisters, they know all the same nuts and apples on their family tree! I look forward to my next step as a grandmother: celebrating Lauren having her own child or children. Her joy will certainly add to my pot of gold. For now, my life is certainly blessed with "girlie" rainbows and gold.

Chapter 16

Urgent Care, Good Care

As I think back over my life and the situations I have lived through, there are times when I wish I had not had to have quite so much "experience." Yes, I know the adage "What doesn't kill you makes you stronger" and I can't claim it's one of my favourite sayings. When people remark about all that I have been through and how I do what I do, I usually say (with a tiny smile on my face), "What's my option?" I know we get to choose how we react to situations and I have chosen to let all the experiences of my life make me stronger. I remember my dad's words when I was young and sickly, "Why not you, Melody?" I guess so, Dad, but... wouldn't it have been nice if somebody else had volunteered to survive then thrive? My chronic poor health, whether in my youth or today, regularly exhausts me physically and mentally.

I feel like I am strong enough. I feel like I have had enough "experiences" in life. As John Lennon once sang, "Life is what happens to you while you're busy making other plans." We cannot choose the events that happen, but we can choose how we deal with them. After you have a transplant of any kind, there is a feeling that you have lived through a lifetime of medical trauma. You limp away from the acute surgical experience (i.e., the experience is lifelong) confident you've had your fair share of tough breaks. You actually expect to live your life with no more medical mishaps, disasters, and bad luck.

As a new organ or tissue recipient, you don't expect other illness to come along. You think you're over the worst parts of your life, and why wouldn't you? You feel like you've been blessed with a precious gift and you're confident life is going to get better and better. I remember after my first transplant thinking smooth sailing and fewer hospital visits were ahead of me. But life loves our plans, doesn't it? Those of us with "gifts of life" inside us still face what others face, especially the long list of catastrophic diseases. Life is just too perfect to be fair, right? Recipients are spared from death for a time but we are not spared from the pain of being human. All 8 billion of us live inside fragile bodies and if you're a transplant recipient, you're pretty much living inside a glass house. Our immune systems are permanently compromised because of the lifelong "anti-rejection" medications we must take. Our white blood cells need constant instruction not to attack the new organ or tissue. Wouldn't it be lovely if we could all receive a "get out of jail card" from these terrible realities? For the majority of us in the organ-and-tissue community, getting cancer is our greatest nightmare. Cancer wrecks particular havoc on our already compromised immune system so when a recipient gets cancer, the stakes are very, very high. A battle of life and death unfolds quickly, aggressively, and brutally. We're four times more likely to develop cancer than "normal" people.

I have been a part of the transplant community for more than 35 years. I have attended the funerals of too many recipients, men, women, and, god help us, children, who've perished because of cancer. I consider the deceased not only cherished friends but heroes who've fought multiple battles. Walking the line between life and death so delicately, makes recipients intuitive about their physical health. You're not paranoid if something is really wrong with you! Any little lump, bump, or change inside or outside my body activates anxiety. For most recipients, when things feel wrong with our body we must answer one question: Do I run immediately to my doctor? Or do I wait and see what happens? I have done both.

A few years after my first transplant, I started being treated for a new affliction: warts. The ghastly growths were mostly on my feet, but some were on my hands. I decided that a few warts wouldn't kill me or get me down. Months of treatments resulted in me befriending all the nurses who "burned" away my warts. You can always find gratitude if you look deeply enough. Of course, there are times when life doesn't hand you a wart, but an actual worry. A growth on my left forearm definitely worried me, especially as the growth started to redden and expand. I rushed to the doctor and guess what? Skin cancer. Bingo! My nightmare and fear realized. The removal left one of the worst scars, caused by more than a dozen stitches. Yet considering the alternative, a scar (which I've reframed as one of my many "beauty marks") is not really a big deal. Like sickness, scars have shaped me into the person I am today.

My final round of skin cancer removals happened more than 15 years ago, on the day I was celebrating my 50th birthday. My special July afternoon in 2006 was spent with a cosmetic surgeon, having growths on my chest and hairline removed. One memory from my birthday party later that day was noticing my chest wound had bled through my blouse. Nothing like having the person being celebrated bleeding all over the place. A new bandage fixed the problem, the party went on, and I was able to thank Shamus, Lauren and April for hosting such a bloody fun party. Thanks and gratitude, as always, to my kids.

I am continually grateful to the medical professionals who've treated me over the years. Weeks before the pandemic hit, I found myself sitting in the waiting room at Urgent Care, a medical facility near where we live, which is open every day from morning until night. People looking for stitches, setting broken bones, and treatment of minor illnesses come here rather than cluttering up the ER downtown. I had taken Koda, our dog, to PetSmart for a bath the day before Lauren was to return from up north in Deer Lake, where she'd been teaching for six months. I'd missed Lauren fiercely and looked forward to celebrating her homecoming. What better way to welcome my daughter home than to present her with our giant, friendly, shaggy, silly dog washed and smelling nice?

While Koda and I waited for the groomer, two more dogs entered the waiting room, causing Koda to get agitated and accidentally claw my left shin. I'm a bleeder. Anyone else would have had a scrape, but me, my medications, and my paper-thin skin? I had a wound. I said patiently and quickly to the staff, "I need paper towel, and lots of it." Blood poured on the floor and, of course, the dogs went wild! While Koda the Shin Cutter had his bubble bath, I drove the five minutes to Urgent Care. I'd refused the offer of an ambulance since I've never loved theatrics or sirens. Even while my leg was bleeding and throbbing, I was feeling thankful; thankful I had access to people who could help me and thankful I would not lose my house or my savings to pay for my healthcare. I also felt grateful for all the chaotic help I received at PetSmart. I doubt those young people will ever forget Koda, the Cute Claw Dog!

If I had had to pay for all the treatments I have undergone in my life, I would either be living in a cardboard box or I'd be dead. Hundreds of thousands, if not millions, of dollars of care. Unfathomable, really. I am so grateful to be Canadian and to have paid into a system that helps millions of Canadians every day. Not only are the big things covered for people (e.g., organ transplants, heart surgery, cancer treatment, baby deliveries) but the tiny things that aren't so small in importance like stitches and staples because of one ridiculous accident or mishap. Or dog. It is incredibly frustrating to have skin this fragile. I do the best I can to be careful, but I seem to continually get into situations which cause me grief. In a span of a couple of weeks I managed to get an abrasion on my right elbow while trying to give my granddaughter a big push on the swing. I once fell up the stairs running to the bathroom, skinning my elbow but bleeding profusely and needing stitches!

But back to that silly dog of mine. Because my skin is so fragile and Koda's claw came into direct contact with my shin, there was not enough skin to stitch together. My medical team decided steri-strips (think of a bandage on steroids) would hold the skin together so I could start healing. Not only did the wound hurt a lot but after three days, there was still blood leaking out of my leg. Like I said, I'm a bleeder! Within a week of the accident at PetSmart, the leg wound was infected, which meant another trip to the doctor, another round of antibiotics, a new specialist, and at-home nurse visits. Oh yes, all this medical care (and inconvenience, I'll admit) because I took my dog for a bath!

I like to think Koda looked ashamed and guilty every time I wrapped my leg compress in a garbage bag when I showered. I'd balance on my good leg while holding my wounded leg over the side of the bathtub in an attempt to keep the compress dry. This particular way of showering was more or less successful, not overly safe, but it was the best I could do. Not all of us are entitled to bubble baths like Koda!

Not to belabour the point or bore you with my clumsiness, but a few other incidents. One day, when I had taken a day off work, I decided to go to (terrible, I try to boycott them) Walmart. On my way into the store, a person rammed into the back of my leg with their shopping cart. Not my doing. Not my fault. Again, I knew right away I was in trouble. Fortunately, I always carry tissue in my purse so once I had staunched the flow of blood, I hobbled to my car and my First Aid kit. (Know thyself). Once again, off to Urgent Care, this time for stitches. I admit, I've developed some anxiety whenever I see shoppers armed with shopping carts!

And Koda's bubble bath days are over. My dog smells just fine.

Chapter 17

Dialysis, Drugs... or Death

Organ donation is miraculous. Being the recipient of not one but two kidneys, this much I know for sure: organ donation changes your life for the better. Even after all these years of advocating for and publicly speaking about organ donation, I am still blown away by the miracle of receiving a heart, lung, or pancreas transplant. The stories I've heard are nothing less than magical and give me faith, again and again, in the future of humanity. We are a generous and gracious species, we really are.

For example, in the case of heart, lung, and/or pancreas donation, the donor likely made the decision to "give the gift of life" while they were alive and well. Death and legacy were only concepts when that donor decided to help their fellow human. For kidney (that's me!), liver, and bone marrow donation, donors can be like my brother Tim, blessed with decades of life after their 100 percent altruistic donation. As you'd guess, living donation demands absolutely clarity around donor motivation. There must be no coercion, no threats, or offers of payment. Whether a donor is deceased or living, I believe organ donation is one of the most beautiful and truly altruistic decisions any of us can make. One donor can save up to eight people. Eight lives whisked away from death's door! And consider the ripple effect, I tell audiences and small groups. You have the potential to save one life and spare that person's family and friends from the devastation of loss and grief. Tissue donation is even more impressive, considering a donor can save up to 75 people!

I love telling people that the oldest organ donor was over 90 years old. Another hero donated tissue and they had just blown out 100 candles on their (last) birthday cake. When I look to the future, I see a world where every man, woman, and child worldwide receives the gift they need to live and prosper. I want no one to get left behind and die needlessly waiting for a new organ or tissue transplant. There are so many problems in the world but transplantation is a problem we can transform into a possibility and a life-affirming "win" for billions of people around the world. Giving all people a shot at health, vitality, and a robust quality of life is possible. I passionately believe that organ donation is one of the most effective (sure, not the sexiest or most comfortable) ways of extending life, sharing love, and giving back.

Despite the miraculous nature of transplantation, there are often side effects due to the number of lifelong medications the recipient must take to ensure that the body's white blood cells do not attack the new intruder, the transplanted organ and/or tissue. As I write this in 2021, most people now understand what life is like after receiving a transplant. Does this sound familiar? We are advised to physically distance from all friends and family. Viruses of all shapes and sizes are potentially lethal to us. And large gatherings are strictly forbidden. Post-transplant life is a lot like lock down life, indeed! After my kidney transplant the only "socializing" I participated in were weekly blood tests that decreased to monthly and then finally to four times a year.

In life there is always a price to pay. I have my health because of organ donation and transplantation. I am forever grateful. But I don't get away unscathed. The price I pay is dealing with the effects of long-term medication use. Each and every day I gobble down about 18 pills that help keep me alive, healthy, and happy. If I'm on antibiotics, guess what? More pills. I feel like I am constantly battling something, but I would not change this routine for the world. My kidney is working and I plan on keeping this organ happy for a long, long time. If taking these medications is how I sustain life, so be it. Of course, I would be happier if there were not so many side effects to the medication, but what are my choices? Live or die. Drugs, dialysis, or death. The choice really is black and white for me and my family. I will always choose life until the day I decide otherwise.

For people who like to be in control, knowing that there is nothing they can do to repair their body is far from comfortable. For those who are impatient, an organ-and-tissue waiting list can feel like torture, mental pain as well as physical pain. Imagine living your life and then suddenly you're told you need a new body part. Trust me, it's a shock facing the reality that you may not survive if you do not receive a new organ. Not only must you face the fact that your body is falling apart and failing, you must also own up to your mortality, and roll the dice too. Depending on your illness, you're at the mercy of finding a compatible living donor or, take a deep breath here, waiting for someone to die so you can live. And just like with any other type of major surgery, going "under the knife" comes with all kinds of inherent risks and threats.

A friend of mine developed heart problems as he aged. He had been healthy and robust until he wasn't. His "engine" needed replacement. I am in awe when I consider such a strange circle of life. Someone dies. That someone made a decision in life to give life. And that gift, in my friend's case, was receiving a new heart from a generous, dead stranger. When I am talking to groups or individuals about organ donation, there is generally some hesitation about actually agreeing to register as a donor. People do not want to think about or talk about their own or their loved one's mortality. Death is not something that most people, especially North Americans, are comfortable talking about. I believe we'd rather talk about money or sex than dying and death! The reality is that we are all going to die some day, hopefully not too soon. If you could have the opportunity to impact someone's life positively (in other words, extend their life by saving it), would you not want to contribute in that way? Isn't organ donation a type of "eternal life" considering your spirit is gone but, like my now healthy friend, your heart continues to beat inside another person's chest?

It saddens me when I meet people incapable of seeing beyond their own death. They view death as "lights out" so there's no impetus to help the living. Yet once we are done with our body, why not let someone else have life and health for as long as possible? Perhaps that's my faith, a blend of religion and spirituality, that lets me see life through this lens. But most people would do just about anything to save the life of someone they love. For me, organ-and-tissue donation is a no-brainer. If I could donate my brain, I would!

There are parts of organ transplantation that hurt my brain. For example, some of the side effects of the medications adversely impact the health of my kidneys. Can you imagine? Did I not receive not one but two new kidneys over the years yet my anti-rejection drugs beat up the very organ the medication is trying to protect? While my brain spins, my bones grow more fragile. Decades of taking prednisone and baby aspirin have escalated my osteoporosis, which I'm pretty sure has led to arthritic pain in my back. Prednisone is also notorious for causing massive weight gain as well as a moon-shaped face but I've been spared those effects. Early on, I made the decision that there was no way I was eating my way through my gift of life, forcing my new kidney(s) to work harder because I wouldn't/couldn't stop eating! I was once asked by a doctor to sit in his waiting room so I could be his "poster girl recipient" for the other transplant recipients, proving that gaining weight and/or becoming obese was not a non-negotiable side effect of taking prednisone. I was touched by the offer, but declined the opportunity. I spend more than enough time at clinics and hospitals so don't feel a need to sign up for even more time there, even if I am being praised and adored for my svelte-skinny figure!

I am skinny and shaky too. There have been times when my hands have shaken so much that I am afraid to put on my mascara. Again, another side effect of medications. I've learned how to avoid gouging my eyes out despite my shaky hands. Plus, I am motivated: this girl can't leave the house without her mascara. Shaky hands also impact my tea drinking. Sometimes I need to hold the cup with both hands to make sure my tea doesn't spill and burn my paper-thin skin. I could go on all day listing side effects so I'll end on this one, which is a real stinker. One lesser side effect post-transplant includes "functional diarrhea," a label that made me laugh the first time my doctor diagnosed me. As far as I am concerned, there is nothing "functional" about five-alarm emergency bathroom breaks!

What a lot of people don't know is that taking tons of prescription medicine is a simpler, kinder solution than the other option. No, not death: dialysis. Organ donor recipients of all stripes detest the term "rejection." And kidney people like me absolutely shake and shiver when we hear the word "dialysis." Living life on dialysis is not a fate worse than death, but the sentence feels like a cruel, unusual, terrible, unfair punishment. Can you tell I don't like dialysis?

Dialysis is an artificial way of cleaning one's blood, which is the traditional function of the kidneys. If your kidneys are weak or failing, your blood and your blood pressure aren't healthy, either.

Hemodialysis carries blood out of the body and into a dialyzer, a machine that cleans the blood of toxins, and then carries the cleaned blood back into the body. Hospital or clinic treatments are scheduled three to five times a week, each treatment is three to four hours long. As I said earlier, dialysis, like ill health in general, erodes quality of life on so many fronts. Peritoneal dialysis is no less invasive or time consuming. A catheter is inserted into the abdomen, so a dialysis solution can leech out toxins and excess fluid. The treatment must happen daily but at least the patient is able to have the procedure done in the comfort and privacy of their home.

In the spring of 2000, my first transplant began to fail after 18 years of more or less perfect functioning. I asked my nephrologist, a kidney specialist, if I was going to lose the kidney and he replied nonchalantly that yes, I probably was. When he saw my horrified expression, he assured me they'd find me a new kidney, which I considered a flippant and inappropriate response. I was well aware that dialysis and death had just entered into the conversation in a very big and scary way. I am not sure why the specialist was so blasé about my bad news. Last I checked, kidneys were not growing on trees.

When I told my brother Tim that his donated kidney was acting up, I joked and asked if he was willing to give me his other kidney. We both smiled sadly. Losing my kidney (formerly Tim's kidney) was going to be a huge loss. I had assumed that my transplant would last me for the rest of my days. I thought my brother's gift of life would stay with me until death. I was married to my kidney, 'til death do us part sort of thing, but the kidney had other plans. I knew I was not interested in doing hemodialysis unless it was the only viable choice. One small mercy was that daily peritoneal dialysis allowed me to stay at home, hooked up to my trusty machine every night for over 18 months. The dialysis machine was keeping me alive, a fact I knew and so did my entire family. We were frightened by the road that lay ahead of me.

My mother and Shamus came forward as potential donors. But doctors determined Mom was too old and Shamus, 21, wasn't a match because of his high blood pressure. My son was devastated by the rejection, which pained me deeply, especially watching him battle shingles shortly after he received the red light from my kidney doctors. I knew that God would provide for me as had always been the case throughout my life. Sure enough, I met someone at church months later, a man named Ernest. We started dating and guess who agreed to be tested, was a match, and wanted to be my donor? Thank you, God. Thank you, Cupid. Three years had passed since I was given the bad news about Tim's kidney. I'd spent the last 18 months on dialysis so Ernest's offer was such a welcome blessing and a profound relief for all of us. By this time, while SARS roared throughout Toronto hospitals (and delayed surgeries like mine), I was in the end stage of renal failure. Time was ticking and the clock was absolutely against me.

In the summer of 2003, I received my new kidney after four hours of surgery. Ernest's surgery, the removal of his kidney, obviously happened before mine. As the nurses walked me into an adjoining surgical room, they directed my vision to a shiny silver box. Inside was my new life: a new kidney. As before, I woke up post-surgery knowing immediately that my body was working better. It is amazing how quickly a healthy kidney transforms one's health from sickly to spectacular. I was up and walking around within hours. True, I did have my friend morphine to help me. Although I was older and wiser, my recovery was even faster than the first transplant. I was discharged within six days and celebrated at home with Ernest, who'd been released days earlier.

My romantic relationship with Ernest lasted another three years. Going our separate ways in no way diminishes my gratitude and appreciation for his gift of life to me. Adequately and thoroughly thanking someone for blessing you with more time on Earth is impossible. Words fail me. But every time I hug a member of my family, I am overwhelmed with gratitude for the people, and the organs, that have kept me here within such a loving circle of life.

Chapter 18

A Shocking Event

In March 2004, Mom was just shy of her 80th birthday. Mom's husband Dudley, my former uncle, was just a year older. While Mom was visiting us in Toronto that early spring, she suffered a life-altering stroke in the middle of the night. Since calling an ambulance did not even cross my mind, I loaded Mom into the car and off we went downtown to the hospital. The staff hurried Mom into a wheelchair and started diagnostic procedures. Mom had a brain bleed on her left side, which explained why the right side of her body was moving slowly and behaving as if partially paralyzed. Mom's speech was slurred too.

Mom was not a big believer in annual physical checkups and had not visited a doctor in many years. I suspect that her blood pressure had become way too high and triggered the brain bleed. It is easy to have 20/20 vision when you're looking backwards and evaluating your choices. Of course, if I had known Mom was having a stroke that night, I would have called 911 immediately and asked for an ambulance. But I didn't. I try not to beat myself up too much after all these years, but showing self-compassion and self-forgiveness is no easy task. You don't know what you don't know. And there's no guarantee an ambulance would have prevented some of the long-term damage Mom carried for years afterwards. The inner chant "If only" and "I should have" is a rabbit hole of painful regret.

Mom's husband flew in from Winnipeg as soon as he could. Dudley was a man of few words so it was hard to know his thoughts. He let his wife visit her kids in Toronto and now she was in hospital. Did he blame Mom's stroke on the evils of visiting Toronto? Did he hold me responsible? We never knew Dudley's true thoughts but he was clear about wanting Mom back where she belonged, with him in Manitoba. I thought Mom should stay in Toronto, a city with world-class medical facilities far superior to those in small town Neepawa, but a daughter's opinion does not carry as much weight as a husband's, I soon discovered. Within weeks I was overruled by both Dudley and my brothers, who all insisted Mom be returned to Manitoba. I knew the men weren't wrong, but it was painful and a real blow to feel that my opinion counted for nothing. I was an adult and had an opinion that was valid and deserved contemplation. But I was also a female and therefore not stable or capable (in their view alone, I assure you) in proposing ideas better than their own. Dudley and my brothers clearly believed they knew what was best for Mom, just by their being male and "heads of households." Frustrating? You bet. In any conversations we had, either just us or with the medical staff at Toronto General, I do not once remember being asked what I thought. As far as my brothers were concerned, I was still their sickly little sister, incapable of making mature, adult decisions or having insightful opinions. I felt like my brothers had put me in a box when I was younger and they did not want to let me out.

Mom was sadly silent as her husband and children attempted to take charge. Given the paralysis on her right side, Mom never walked or talked properly ever again. I cry as I write that. Mom spent the rest of her life in a wheelchair. With physiotherapy, started in Toronto and maintained (thankfully!) in Neepawa, Mom was able to push herself around in a tall walker. Due to the lack of strength on her right side, she needed the support of the armrests on the walker to keep her upright. She had been a right-handed person and now needed to figure out how to use her left hand. Not an easy task but one she ultimately conquered. Mom's speech also remained severely impacted. Even with therapy, she often mixed up her pronouns, sometimes saying "she" for Shamus and "he" for Lauren. To this day I am thankful Mom's stroke did not sever our connection. We could still communicate. I always eventually figured out what she needed, what she wanted, and what she was trying to say. For that, I am grateful. A small mercy during a difficult and sad time.

In retrospect, Mom's stroke was a real growing experience for me. Not only did I decide I was no longer going to be insulted and ignored by my brothers, I also committed to visiting Mom regularly, no matter what. No one, and I mean no one, was going to keep me away from my mother. My brothers "let me" fly Mom home to Dudley, our flight there made smoother thanks to the help and accompaniment of my niece, who is a nurse. As planned, we were met in Winnipeg by an ambulance that transported Mom to Neepawa's tiny hospital, a gruelling two-hour trip after an uncomfortable two-hour flight. I was relieved when I discovered that Mom was relocated to Brandon, a larger community about an hour outside Neepawa, that had a stroke recovery program. Sure, Brandon was not Toronto but at least Mom was not stranded alone with Dudley receiving zero therapy or stuck in Neepawa's bone-basic hospital. Mom did well in Brandon, receiving the help and support she desperately needed. As Mom progressed and became stronger, I realized that staying in Toronto had not been the only viable option, which made me feel less panicked about Mom being so sick and so far away.

Once Mom was home with Dudley, a nurse visited her every day, helping with showering and dressing, and offering a social outlet that Mom desperately missed. Mom's diminished health cut her off from her favourite and most meaningful social interactions. She was no longer able to go to church, attend Bible study or visit friends. When I sometimes thought Mom's friends had deserted her, I had to remind myself that those old ladies weren't spring chickens either! There were a few (younger) people who still came to visit and I was always so grateful to hear about these visitors from Mom. One regular visitor was the church organist and school music teacher. This lovely lady would bring her portable keyboard and play all the hymns Mom loved. The music always brought a smile to her face. Like mother like daughter, indeed.

I flew to Winnipeg as often as I could get away, usually every six to eight weeks. The trips to Manitoba were tiring but necessary. One year, I made a trip in mid-May. When I left Toronto, it was 30 degrees. When I arrived in Winnipeg, there had been a blizzard the night before! What a huge country we call home. Because of the snowstorm, the highway to Brandon was closed for over 24 hours. The delay meant I would have less time to visit with Mom. Once the highway reopened, I began my journey to Brandon. A car trip that usually took two hours took four (snowy, dangerous) hours! More time spent away from my mom.

I was so grateful that I had already had my second transplant and, as such, was as healthy and strong as I could be. Since Mom was limited in her speech, it was hard to really know how she was doing by just having a conversation on the phone. By visiting in-person, I was able to assess for myself how she was doing: mentally, physically, and emotionally. Her speech was more understandable, which allowed her to engage in short simple conversations if people were patient and understanding.

Mom was always financially generous with me. Her cheque-writing was now done by her left hand since her right hand was paralyzed. I was always amazed by how much my mother's beautiful handwriting had been changed by the stroke. Every time, no matter how I resisted, Mom always gave me a cheque that covered more than my travel expenses, which she insisted on paying, including my flight and car rental. We both enjoyed the freedom of having a car. We'd go for drives in the country and sometimes go out for dinner, just the two of us. Mom would always order liver and onions, one of her all-time favourite meals.

As the months and years passed, I knew that Dudley and my brothers were convinced that I was taking advantage of Mom's generosity. Every time she wrote me a cheque, I felt a little uncomfortable and made sure I thanked her profusely. She would say, "I have it, you need it." This is a comment Lauren and I say to one another when it comes to finances. I'm proud that Lauren and I are breaking a dysfunctional family legacy that insisted we never directly talk about difficult subjects, money being one of the biggest. My mother's husband once did question me about some chequebook entries and made it clear that he was watching and feeling resentful. My response was cold and, worse, angry and hurt. I've never been a fan of confrontation so my cold silence seemed preferable to a nasty scene.

Although our roles had been reversed suddenly and tragically, I was grateful to take care of my mother. I had the energy and the health to look after someone I desperately loved and wanted to protect and cherish. I read to Mom, hosted harp concerts for her, cut her nails, talked to her, brushed her hair, read the Bible to her, and prayed with her. I wouldn't change a single second of all that time I spent with Mom. We were happy, both of us, when we were together. It may have looked like I was taking care of her, acting like a caregiver more than a daughter, but life is a two-way street. Mom was taking care of me too. We all need our mothers. That reality doesn't change irrespective of how old you are. Our quiet visits made me feel like I was somehow making the world kinder and better, and more fair, by taking care of Mom.

The house where Mom and Dudley lived had a screened-in porch. Weather permitting, we would have our afternoon tea out on the porch after we'd both had our post-lunch afternoon naps. As we sipped our tea, we could hear the birds, sometimes catching sight of a hummingbird as it flitted by. Mom and I would chat or we would sit in amiable silence. Those porch afternoons are some of my most cherished memories of my mother. From the comfort of the porch, we'd also admire her garden's flowers, bursts of blooms in the ground and inside cracked but charming pots. Our favourite flowers were the pansies, their flower faces smiling up at you. The origin of "pansy" is the French word "penser," to think about or remember. When I see pansies today, I always think of Mom. And I always remember those afternoons on the porch when life was broken but exceptionally beautiful too.

Chapter 19

Stroke of Insight

Whenever I visited Mom in Manitoba, Dudley's presence added a tremendous amount of tension to the household. While visiting in August 2004, approximately five months after Mom's stroke, Dudley informed me I was unwelcome in his home. Mom likely overheard this terrible announcement, so I attempted to remain civil and calm. I understood that I was visiting his house, but this was the home of my best friend, my mother, and I was dedicated to her physical and mental well-being. I'd always known Dudley had never liked me, but I was never sure why. Even when he was married to my aunt, my mother's sister, I could tell I was not his favourite person.

Perhaps Dudley was jealous of the relationship Mom and I had. Yet our closeness must not have come as a surprise. He knew mother and daughter were close long before their marriage. His insistence that Mom move back to Manitoba after her stroke might have fostered hope in him that he'd never have to see me again. An absolutely incorrect, and foolish, assumption. My brothers and I were dedicated to Mom, so were all her grandchildren. I knew no one, especially a jealous and petty man, would stop me from seeing and caring for my mom. There was no way Mom would be separated from those who loved her, not on my watch.

I felt so sorry for Mom on a number of levels. She was married to Dudley, she was injured because of a stroke, and now she'd overheard her husband of 13 years tell her daughter she was forbidden to visit. My poor mother really believed that Dudley would keep me away. She'd listened to the whole terrible conversation from the prison of her wheelchair. I get choked up as I write that. Mom was frail and wounded, but strong. She'd remained quiet, unable to speak clearly or easily, but I know she had plenty to say. Maybe even to scream. As soon as I ended the conversation with Dudley, I returned to the living room. Mom began to cry and I refused to. I reassured her that I would come to see her as often as I could regardless of what Dudley said or tried to do. "Not to worry, Mom. We'll figure something out. No one is keeping me from you. No one."

In the end and as promised, I continued my visits. When I arrived on their doorstep, Dudley would leave immediately and stay with one of his children from his first marriage. One son lived in Portage la Prairie, about an hour away, and his daughter lived two hours away in Winnipeg. Good. I am confident his children enjoyed their father's company. Mom and I enjoyed his absence. Having the house all to ourselves was wonderful. There was no tension, only relief and joy that we were reunited at last. We could talk as we wanted, listen to music as loud as we liked, and eat when and whatever we wished. A type of mother-daughter "girls' weekend." There was such relaxation in being unobserved and free from Dudley's negativity.

There was no denying that I had become my mother's caregiver. I was no longer sickly and small, yet Mom was both of those things now. Her spirit remained as large as ever. Mom's heart was open wide, her mind always ready for new ideas and experiences. Taking care of her felt like benevolent, loving payback. Growing up, Mom had always been there for me whether I was burdened with a physical crisis or a crisis of the heart. During this time with Mom, my health was stronger than it had been in decades. I am always grateful for my good health but looking back on those years with Mom, I am particularly grateful. Every day with Mom out on that porch was a gift. There is never a guarantee of how long good health will last. I knew that sad unfair reality more than most people. Every time I was in Manitoba taking care of Mom, I felt an overwhelming appreciation for each and every one of my organs, especially that kidney of mine!

In the end, I believe even Dudley started to look forward to my visits. He was Mom's main caregiver and his visits away must have felt like a reprieve. He took good care of Mom, providing for her physical needs, but I believe he was never able to feed her soul or her spirit. The house was a beautiful abode, but I don't believe it was ever a joyful home. Dudley never thought to read to Mom or talk about anything other than the weather or maybe something that was on the news. I believe living a lifetime in rural Manitoba limited his capacity for spiritual and intellectual conversation. Dudley was a hardworking man and overall a good man. He was a successful and profitable farmer yet bridging the gap between nature and God eluded him. Her husband's lack of religious or spiritual faith isolated my mother even further. She'd always had a personal relationship with God, which I'm confident she would have liked to share with her husband. You know what they say, a family that prays together, stays together.

Mom's relationship with God was dynamic and changed as she grew older. After her stroke, she was very angry with God. Rather than being delivered to a peaceful afterlife, Mom was spared to face a life of limitation and lacking a significant amount of joy and independence. Being in a hospital bed when you were promised heaven could make even the most faithful furious. I appreciated how Mom felt comfortable letting me know, slowly and painstakingly because of her stuttered speech, just how betrayed she felt. I cannot really blame her and I was relieved when she and God reunited. I am confident my mother missed her relationship with God, and I am equally confident God missed my mother. Amazing to think the two of them are now together but separate from me.

While Mom slowly rebuilt a loving relationship with her circumstance and her faith, I came to the conclusion that I was unhappily married and needed to leave so I could survive. Thriving would come later. Mom and I regularly talked about our marriages. Dudley was proving a partner who offered little passion or companionship which was similar to the reality Bob and I were living. Unlike myself, Mom didn't dare even contemplate leaving her marriage. She knew the pain and humiliation of heartbreak (remember, my father had left her) so she refused to inflict the same pain on her second husband. Plus, Mom was elderly and sickly. No one ever said life was fair.

As Mom and I strategized about how to make ourselves happier, I realized she was encouraging me to have the strength to do what I needed to do. She had decided to stay in her marriage, but that did not mean that I had to suffer a similar fate. I wanted a bigger, better, happier life. So did my mother but it was I who'd make the changes to turn that dream into a reality. Feeling like I had her approval was not essential for me to move on with my life. But I drew strength knowing that no matter what my marital decision, my mother would love and support me. As she always had. Obviously conversations about marriages and men never happened when Lauren visited Mom with me.

Lauren and her grandmother had a special relationship, rooted in all the quality time they had spent together when Lauren was growing up. Whenever Mom had visited Toronto, she'd share a room with Lauren, the two of them staying up late and giggling like little girls. Mom loved to hear Lauren play the piano, which she did often, especially for her Granny. Just like years before in Toronto, when Lauren and I visited Mom in Manitoba, we'd include her in all our antics and shenanigans. Whether it was singing as we baked cookies or taking long walks in the sunshine, Mom was "one of the gang." We involved her in anything and everything we could. Our intention was always to inspire Mom to feel that she was respected, fully capable, and always the centre of our loving attention.

Once or twice Shamus and April accompanied me to Manitoba. April had not met Mom before she had her stroke, but the two women communicated simply and warmly. I remember smiling and laughing when Mom told me that April was a "keeper." Mom enjoyed having people visit, although communicating post-stroke took its toll on her. She'd be vibrant for a bit followed by a lie down or lengthy nap. In many ways, Mom reminded me of when I was young: good days and bad days, energy versus no energy. But Mom was more gracious about her health, less impatient than my younger self. Obviously, Mom was wiser, a positive consequence of living years with an open and courageous heart.

For me and Mom, summertime meant birthday time. Hers was in June and mine was in July. Of course, being together for our birthdays was always special but increasingly difficult with distance and Dudley between us. Yet for Mom's 87th birthday, the stars aligned. Mary, one of my mother's lifelong friends, joined me on my trip to the Prairies. The three of us spent days enjoying the warm June weather, the delicious tea, and the storytelling. As in life, none of us knew that Mom's special birthday would in fact be her last. A month later, when Lauren and I headed out to Manitoba again to celebrate my 55th birthday, our party consisted of eating ice cream cake and wondering if the three of us would ever be with each other again. As parents age and grow ill, goodbyes are transformed into excruciating events. Every time I said goodbye to Mom, I did my best to keep a brave face until I was sure Mom couldn't see me. With Lauren present, I was especially tough. I could not contemplate never seeing my mother again. After my birthday celebration, and with Lauren beside me in the car, we drove away, watching my mother's fading figure waving weakly from the porch. Unlike previous years I didn't drive away for a kilometre or two, pull the car over, and hysterically cry about leaving my mother behind. We pay a heavy heart tax loving people we know we're destined to lose. My goodness, life can be such a beautiful and heart-wrenching conundrum.

Mom had taught me a lot about dying and death long before she grew old and ill. When she was still married to my father and a much younger woman, Mom was involved with Dying with Dignity, a human-rights charity aimed at giving Canadians more end-of-life rights. Mom believed fully in the sanctity of life while simultaneously seeing death as a process that deserved dignity and self-determination. When Mom began to decline, I had the awful feeling that she would ask me to help her pass from this world to the next. I couldn't fathom what I'd be expected to do. My mother represented life and everything that made life worth living. Fortunately, life never demanded that I actively participate in my mother's dying. Another small mercy.

When her time was over on this earth, Mom left us. Mom died in hospital. She died in Manitoba. None of her children were there. Mom did not have her teeth in and her positioning looked odd and uncomfortable.

I believe Mom did not die with as much dignity and self-determination as she would have liked. Another cruel injustice that Mom advocated for years for the dying and when it was her time, so many of her wishes were left unfulfilled. Tim and I arrived 30 minutes too late; Mom had exhaled her last breath. This gracious woman's suffering was finally over. Our suffering and grief began. Of course, I was devastated when Mom died. But my mom had been gone, for the most part, for more than seven years because of the stroke. That brain bleed had stolen so much from her, her children, and her grandchildren. She was not the mom who had read "Anne of Green Gables" to me. Nor was she the mom who had baked shortbread and fruitcake. Mom was so cruelly diminished from the woman she had been, the mother who raised us. I can still feel vapour trails of anger about the unfairness of it all. But who am I to judge? Who am I to complain? Despite the physical hardships and communication gaps, Mom remained the same loving and caring woman she'd always been. Her spirit remained just as bright and loving. Mom was always there for me and always concerned about my well being. My mother "mothered" me right to her final day on Earth, and I am grateful for that and to her. It's how I plan on mothering my children and grandchildren, right to the end. I pledge this right now: until my dying breath, those I love will know that I love them.

With Mom's death there would be no more "I love you" whispered into ears. No more messages left on my phone saying she was calling to see how I was doing. I like to believe that Mom died peacefully, confident in the lives stretching out before each of her children, grateful her children could move forward without her. I sadly smile at the thought of Mom making those first few steps into the afterlife, free of problems and pain. I am confident Heaven was happy to welcome her. I am grateful she had as much fun and feistiness in this fight called life as she could. I could not have asked for a better mother and better friend.

With Mom gone from the world, I worried that I might be less of a person or that there would be less love and joy in my life. I moved beyond those fears, realizing that Mom is always with me. I will never be alone. With first Dad gone then Mom, I had to look at the new reality that I would never have parents again. As I was then, I am now: an orphan. I feel strongly that our deceased loved ones are around us, watching over us, making sure we are protected and never alone. One of these spirits is my mom and my dad is close by as well. I suppose in a way then they are still parenting me but from another dimension and in deeply loving and peaceful ways.

Writing about my mom is difficult. The love I feel for her has not been diminished by her death. Today I look at her life and our relationship through the eyes of love and compassion. The more we love, the more opportunity grief has to break us down so our hearts are broken wide open.

Chapter 20

A Week in My Life, Honest

The following is a snapshot of a week I just survived.

Monday. The car dies in the Tim Horton's drive-through. Lauren pushes the car so we're out of the way and not blocking anyone else from picking up their coffees. Minutes later, the stalled car mysteriously roars to life.

Tuesday. The car dies again when I am at the osteopath. Fortunately, I have a CAA membership. I call them and they're coming. The car starts after I make the call. Of course, it does!

Wednesday. There's pain around my bellybutton. Is it something or nothing? My GP orders an immediate ultrasound. But the car is at the mechanic. I spend seven hours at Urgent Care.

Thursday. I have an incarcerated umbilical hernia. Of course I do! Hernias are common in obese people (not me), women who've had multiple pregnancies (not me), and those with chronic coughs (not me). CT scan means more hours of waiting, waiting, waiting.

Friday. The hernia needs surgery. Not now but soon. More good news? The mechanic has sent a bill but no diagnosis. There's nothing wrong with the car. What I would give for a doctor to say that about my vehicle/body! I meet friends for a luncheon, enjoying the sunshine and lakeside breeze.

Saturday. Lauren and I are walking the dog. We chat with our nice basement neighbour. He is moving out because the landlord's ex-wife is moving in. She has three young children, all of them loud and rambunctious. Lauren and I see a move in our future. I hope the car keeps moving too.

That week I just survived? That's just a few months from a global pandemic hitting daily life. We moved just before lock down life decimated Toronto (and the world). The timing of our move was miraculous and, as always, I am grateful.

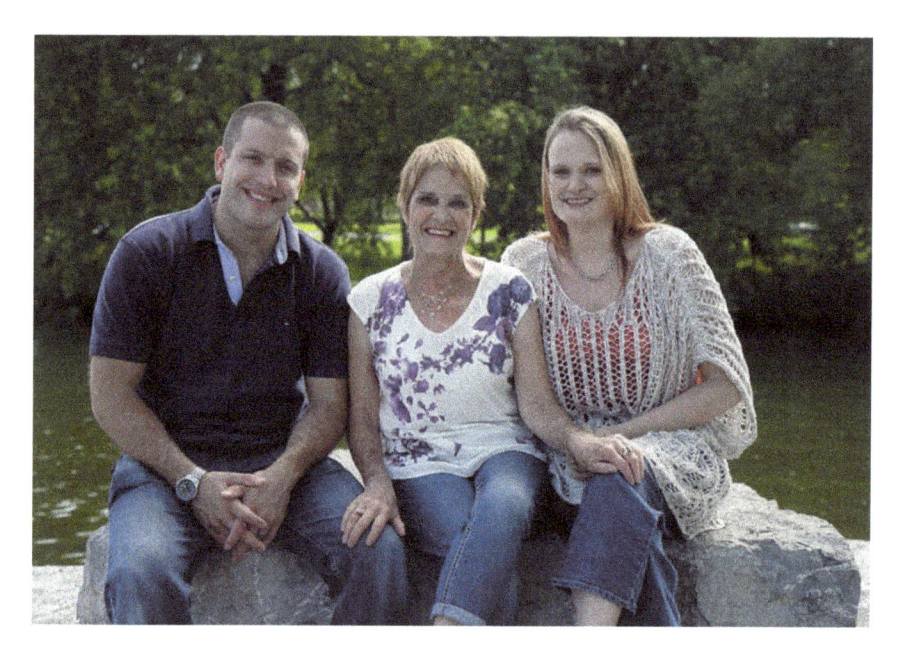

Shamus, me, Lauren, summer 2015

Chapter 21

Where Am I Now?

It has been 36 years since I had my first kidney transplant, a lifetime really. There has been lots of water under the proverbial bridge. There has been hell and there has been high water, but I'm still floating and treading water as best I can.

A recap of my life so far. Shamus is born in 1982; first transplant 1983: David dies in 1984; Shamus's dad and I go our separate ways in 1986; I start dating Bob in at the beginning of 1987; Lauren is born in 1988; Bob and I get married in 1990; I compete in the 1993 Transplant Games in Vancouver and the 1997 Games in Australia; Dad dies in 2000; Bob and I separate in 2001; I begin dialysis in 2002; second kidney transplant happens in 2003 (during SARS); I have a heart attack in January 2009; Shamus and April are married in 2010; Mom dies in 2011; Emma is born in 2012, Lauren graduates with a BFA from York University in 2012; Lily is born in 2014; Lauren receives her Bachelor of Education in 2014; Lauren completes her Masters in Education in 2022. Throw in a couple of rounds of diverticulitis in 2013 and 2014, and a few skin cancer removals. A ton of happy memories, laughs, and some tears. Voila, my life, folks! For the most part.

Throughout all this "stuff," the good, the bad, the ugly plus the spectacular and sorrowful, gratitude trumps everything. I am alive and reasonably well. Every day is a gift. Getting up each morning is truly wonderful. Even when there are tough issues that need to be dealt with, life is good and life is short. Life is not long. I want to make the most of my time here on Earth. Admittedly, these days I find myself spending more time on the couch than I'd prefer. I am definitely not thrilled by this development, as if my quality of life has regressed, which is related to the onset of osteoporosis/osteoarthritis in my back. That sickly little girl stranded on the couch, staring out at the neighbourhood kids playing in the street, remains a wounded side of me. When I am sick, I feel young and vulnerable even though I now qualify as not young and still borderline fragile. I am glad that I am retired and I can listen to my body and give it what it seems to need, such as deep rest and peaceful thoughts. Impatience is not allowed on the couch with me. It's frustrating and more than demoralizing when I am unable to live my life as I wish. Of course, as I reread and rewrite this passage, I am reminded that COVID shifted everyone's life "to the couch" in a way. Sadly, billions of people know what it feels like to have their lives roll off track and crash.

I'm grateful I'm still able to get physical relief despite Toronto's revolving, never-ending lock downs. My osteopath really alleviates the discomfort in my body as well as my mood. Osteopathy was something that I knew nothing about until I met Katharine, a lovely osteopath who had me hooked after just one session of gently manipulating my muscle tissues and bones. Immediate pain relief without drugs was a dream come true. To be released out of suffering and pain is divine, so it's appropriate that Katharine's office is in our church! I may wince and wobble my way onto Katharine's table but within 20 minutes of her magic, I am pain free, walking, and raring to go!

I believe relief is an underrated emotion. Imagine the feeling of finding your lost phone or wallet. Or how about when your kid disappears for a few minutes at the store? Relief is delicious. What tastes bitter and makes life hard? Thinking we're in control. Perhaps I'm delusional but I am not a "control freak." I pity those alpha-people, I really do. Control freaks must feel in charge or they're unhappy and uneasy, prone to lash out and freak out. Having control over my body and my quality of life was taken from me at an early age. My physical well-being and vitality were uncontrollable and random. What I did figure out at a young age, and what I've tried my very best to teach and model to my children, is that sometimes the only choice we have is how we choose to respond to challenges. We can choose to respond thoughtfully and respectfully rather than instinctively spewing a reaction while pressing "panic" inside ourselves and others.

Giving up control while remaining in command of my focus, choices, and mood has been my life's work. Continuing on with grace and kindness is a test of courage and strength. Irrespective of how I might feel physically, every day I really do make an effort to ensure I am doing the best I can with my life. Without physical control, emotional and spiritual maturity are my foundations. They're what make me a better mother, grandmother, and friend. Lack of control has given me the gift of resilience. I am able to bounce back from any given situation, whether it is a broken relationship or another new illness.

I remember dropping off Shamus at Queen's University. My son had chosen to study drama. (Because his mother is dramatic? Who knows!) On the drive back from Kingston, Lauren asked if I had any regrets about my life choices. I answered with a resounding "No, nope, nada." In my opinion, regrets are a waste of time. There is nothing you can do about things that have already happened. I explained to Lauren that there had been things I would have taken a pass on (e.g., being sickly, Mom having a stroke) if I'd been given a choice, but there was no choice but forward. You play the cards you're dealt. Everything that has happened to me has made me the person I am today. And I am okay with who I am. And you know what? I like saying that, that I like who I am.

It's my job to like me not other people's. When I look in the mirror, I love the woman I see. She's a good woman and she's doing her best. I show love and I receive love. My life is good. Sure, even though I feel like I have been to hell and back more than once, I want no pity. From anyone. This has been my life and I have accepted my life, warts and all. I make the best of whatever comes along and I hope those I love follow suit. Life is meant to be lived and cherished. Your life is not intended to be fought against and complained about. Life really is about love.

Resilience has given me plenty of self-confidence, a lot of humour. I realize my laugh is bigger than my body, and I love that. I believe God always has a helping hand in my life. And He will not give me more than I can handle. I know I am a good person to know. I am kind, understanding, altruistic, and have a sharp sense of humour. If people choose not to like me, that's okay. That's their free will and their choice, and their loss too. I'm blessed with family and friends who see the very best in me. Those are my people. The people who love me are a deep well of strength and joy in my life, especially when my days get wild or dark with all that I am unable to control.

Chapter 22

Wanting the Last Word: COVID-19

Once you've had a transplant, you're at a greater risk of getting sick. Germs are not your friends. The medication you take lowers your immune system so your new organ is not attacked. Life post-transplant is definitely a balancing act between medication that protects your new organ and natural immunity that can battle whatever is going around. Working in education for 25 years showed me, especially during flu season, just how well my body could battle germs. As we all know, kids are little adorable germ magnets. Whether it's the copious snot from their stuffy noses or throwing up on a desk (always a favourite for teacher and students!), kids share and spread the wildest things!

In the early spring of 2020, the world went completely crazy. You know what I'm talking about. January 2020 in Toronto was as slate grey and cold as ever. Nothing unusual. We celebrated Lauren's 32nd birthday on the 2nd of January. Christmas had been action packed and joyful, and quieter days were welcome. Looking back, we took so much for granted. We were together. We were hugging and kissing. We were eating and being merry. And none of us was masked or fearful. My goodness, how life changes so quickly. As January progressed, we started hearing about a new super virus causing havoc in China and other parts of Asia. Still nothing for us to worry about in North America. Right? So wrong.

By the end of January, confirmed COVID-19 cases were being reported across China. Before February arrived, the first case was reported in Canada, in Toronto no less, my beautiful and beloved city. The World Health Organization (WHO) declared a Public Health Emergency of International Concern. We were warned that what was happening in China posed a public health risk to other countries and the WHO demanded a coordinated international response. Did Canada really listen? No.

While the world spun off its axis and into turmoil, Lauren and I were blissfully unaware. Like the majority of Canadians, my family and I had no idea how quickly life would change, shut down, be restricted, and basically stop. When looking back on traumatic events, it's funny what you remember. I recall that I'd promised Lauren a spa weekend. I remember that our move was scheduled for early March. And I still toast the fact that we did not wait for joy! Rather than postponing the spa weekend until after we'd moved, we went away mid-February. You just never know when you're having good luck! Looking back, all of us were still so oblivious of what was ahead. To think that after that spa weekend and moving into our new home, we'd be stepping into months and months of restrictions and lock downs. If we had known half of what was to come, I am sure Lauren and I would have enjoyed our time away even more.

Remember those days? The freedom to go from a lovely facial to the cool pool to hot sauna and steam room. All without practising social distancing or wearing a mask! Being away was wonderful. We were both relaxed and rejuvenated when we arrived home. We had just less than three weeks to finish packing up the house and take possession of our new home in mid-March, March 10th to be exact. And the next day, on March 11th, do you remember what happened? Do you remember what you were doing March 11th? I sure do. On the first day inside our new home, the WHO declared COVID-19 a global pandemic. The Canadian Government was suggesting that you not travel and if you were already away that you needed to "come home now" as soon as you could. There was talk that the US/Canada border would close. Unbeknownst to us at the time, international flights continued to arrive into Pearson Airport and every other major Canadian airport without any kind of passenger screening. For almost a year.

It's so hard to wrap your head around the whole situation: what happened then, what happened throughout, and what continues to unfold almost two years later. Our entire world has changed. What did all those initial terrifying announcements mean to me and my family? Not much really. No one really knew what a pandemic was but we were confident we'd be inconvenienced for a couple of weeks. Nothing more. This "pandemic" was just a blip, an inconvenience, almost a novelty, really. And of course we believed the government knew what it was doing and only had our best interests at heart. Life until the middle of March was lovingly normal. April and Lauren were teaching, Emma and Lily were attending school, Shamus was working from home. As for me? I was looking forward to moving into a brighter, quieter home with my daughter. I felt like we were changing our lives and indeed we were. But the world had different plans about just how much our lives would change and shrink. Within days of our move, Toronto went into its first two-week lock down so we could all work together to "flatten the curve." More lock downs would come, most extending for months. Toronto at one point was the most locked-down city on the continent. There was so much uncertainty in those first few weeks about how to live and how to keep your family safe. Around the world, lives were destined to become smaller and smaller. We were told not only as a family but as a country and entire global community that we were to leave our homes only when absolutely necessary. Suddenly going to the doctor, picking up medications at the pharmacy, visiting a grieving friend, or grocery shopping in-person became a matter of "do I or don't I?"

There were mixed messages too. March Break 2020 still happened, a week off for all the school kids and teachers. A beloved springtime tradition for millions of Canadians is to head south for sunshine. (Remember those days? International travel!) Shamus and April and the girls were travelling to Cuba for March Break. What to do? If they went, they would need to quarantine for 14 days upon their arrival home. The day before leaving for Cuba, we gathered at East Side Mario's to celebrate

Lily's sixth birthday. The celebration felt distracted and scattered. Shamus and April were conflicted about whether to go to Cuba or cancel their trip. I was doing my best to keep my mouth shut. No one had asked for my input. In my heart I wanted them to cancel their vacation. Having my son and his family here was more reassuring than having them thousands of miles away. What would happen if they were not able to get home? What if they grew seriously ill while in Cuba?! What if all borders closed and we had to fight to bring my family back to the safety of Canada?

Shamus and April eventually announced that they would fly to Cuba and play the odds. If they saw any indication that international borders were closing, they'd come home immediately. I almost wept when I heard Shamus's voice, telling me they were home safe and sound. Despite their vacation being far from perfect, both Shamus and April had remained anxious about travel restrictions and the possibility of the girls catching COVID, Shamus admitted the sun and beach had lifted their winter-tired spirits.

Spring unfolded with more and more news and medical directives about how to "flatten the curve" across Canada and the world. We were told we were saving lives by staying home. If we left our homes, we were assured, we were risking our lives and the lives of our most vulnerable. A terrible joke went around that each time you went out, you were potentially "killing Gramma." I never developed a lot of humour or wit around COVID. I felt too much like Gramma: vulnerable, older, and sickly. I didn't like where I stood in the pandemic pecking order because I was right up front!

The government implemented bylaws that would fine people for congregating in groups. Church services were cancelled, live theatres went dark, movies shut down. There was no place to go other than the grocery store, drug store, or to pick up food from a restaurant. Lots of independently-owned establishments, beautiful family-run businesses, closed temporarily and later the majority of them closed permanently. Restrictions were changing the landscapes of our communities, cultures, and country. Lauren and I watched from inside our living room. We went on a news diet at one point as the predictions and stories were so dire, especially the criminal negligence happening at long-term care homes.

There were bright spots. While Shamus and April were in Cuba, one of their friends reached out to see if there was anything Lauren and I needed from the grocery store. Lauren was not leaving the house since she was terrified of bringing home germs to me. We both knew I was immune compromised. If I ever stepped into the ring with COVID, I would lose. Knockout.

I was touched by the thoughtfulness of Shamus and April's friend. I figured accepting help or asking for help with groceries would be a one-time event, something that would not be required by the time Shamus and his family returned from Cuba. Wrong! Almost two years later, Lauren and I are pros at ordering all our groceries online. Starting in the spring and well into summer, Lauren and I were only leaving the house for walks and car rides to keep ourselves active and engaged with splashes of new sceneries more interesting than the four walls of our home.

As spring and warm weather finally arrived in Toronto, I needed to get blood work done. Not only did I need to get tests done for the transplant clinic, but my GP wanted to check my thyroid and sodium levels. I was not looking forward to going out. Lauren was anxious too. We'd become house hermits and going out had become a source of stress and anxiety. I refused to have Lauren accompany me. Better one of us brave the elements than our entire tiny household. The day I went out for my blood tests happened to be a particularly windy day. Since I am rather on the small size, the wind blows me around. My brothers called me "Beach Ball" when we were growing up, so it's ironic that at 64 years old, I still consider myself a "big girl." Yet I know in my heart of hearts I'm super tiny, bordering on frail. When it's windy, I like to say I need rocks in my socks to keep from flying away! Sadly, that morning I didn't have my usual sense of humour. I felt nervous and wished I could just hunker down at home with Lauren until this whole pandemic "thing" passed. If only! (Remember when we all thought the pandemic would end within a few weeks and life would just return to normal?)

I left the house for the clinic with plenty of time. I parked the car across from the building and before getting out of the car, I donned my mask. Not only did the wind blow me around, the mask made it extra hard to breathe. By the time I made it inside the clinic, I could hardly speak. I was winded. And the irony was not lost on me. But I didn't smile about it. Plus, no one could see my face anyway! I had decided to keep my winter gloves on, not sit down, and not touch anything while I waited. Since I had an appointment, I hoped I would not have to wait long. As 20 minutes dragged into more than half an hour, and with a mask causing me to almost hyperventilate, I felt angry and impatient. Here I was in a place I never wanted to be, a clinic packed with potentially sick people during a pandemic. I managed my anger and self-pity as best as I could while I waited and waited some more.

As soon as I was home, I put all my clothes into a bag that went immediately into the washing machine. I headed for the shower and washed from head to toe. Taking all these precautions did seem a little over the top but better too much than not enough. I was exhausted for the rest of the day. The physical outing played a part, but my energy was especially depleted by the emotional toll of feeling afraid and being surrounded by frightened people. Looking back, I'm surprised I didn't have myself a big ole ugly cry in the shower. Maybe I did but blocked it out.

After about two months full time at home, things were becoming tedious. At first home life didn't seem too bad. Yes, we were inside but the weather was not great, cold and damp lots of days. As time went by and one week bled into another, life grew blurry and dreary. Another week and another. More groceries online. It was always exciting when we knew there was a delivery coming. A new face! Someone else for the dog to bark at! One thing that bothered me then was Lauren's refusal to allow our local piano tuner into the house to look at our beautiful baby grand piano. The piano needed more than tuning, true, since it's over 100 years old. But what a shame, I thought, to consider how the piano sat unplayed and unloved day after day in our basement. During a time like this in history, wouldn't it be wonderful if Lauren could play not just for her own enjoyment but mine too? Playing the piano was a beautiful way of releasing stress and honing my daughter's God-given talent. I even believed our neighbours would love the sounds of Lauren sharing her passion and creativity.

Happily, that Christmas "Santa" gifted Lauren a complimentary piano tuning and another for her January birthday too. Perhaps we've all grown stronger under these restrictions, more resilient, and willing to practise self-care. Lauren agreed to allow the piano tuner to come to the house so at last, gorgeous piano music was heard in our home every day. At times I am overwhelmed with gratitude and pride listening to the emotion coming down through Lauren's fingers onto the keys and into our tiny world. I know how therapeutic piano playing is for Lauren, the music offering both pleasure and escape. We are currently working on fixing up her cello. Once it is in good shape again, we plan to do some harp-and-cello duets.

These days I've started practising French using Duolingo, a phone app. I spend 30 to 60 minutes a day studying and talking to myself in French, like an official crazy person. Then there's my guitar playing, which I first started when I retired. During the 2020 lock down, I figured I had no excuse not to play and improve since I certainly had the time. Rather than watching Netflix and rotting my brain, I enjoyed the guitar lessons I picked my way through, growing increasingly comfortable with video calls and showing off my guitar playing to my virtual teacher. My personal guitar guru is very kind, patient, and looks a little bit like me, which isn't surprising since my teacher is my son. Shamus is an accomplished guitarist and our time together, even virtually and with my bad guitar playing as a soundtrack, was time well spent during the pandemic. As I look back and list what I did most days, I realize how full my days were. There was even a daily workout I incorporated into my routine! None of those "COVID curves" for me although I realize I could afford to gain a pound or 12.

Today Lauren and I still go out for walks, but we've developed a new habit. We immediately cross the street when we encounter fellow walkers. I stay away from people now, intentionally avoiding them. For a friendly, chatty person like me, who's blessed to live in a safe and welcoming neighbourhood, social distancing hurts my heart. I miss people and I like to think people miss me.

At least now we're able to see Shamus, April, Emma, and Lily in person. For so long we only saw each other from afar, over video, or through the window. No hugs, no cuddles, no snuggles, so hard. I was delighted when Lauren chose to read to her nieces using FaceTime. Not even a pandemic could keep the girlies' ant/auntie away from marching in and spreading love and literature.

The first draft of this memoir was around Day 147 of lock down. I remember writing about wishing I could get a haircut, enjoy a manicure and pedicure, scoot out to the store for a last-minute ingredient without fear or a mask. Even now in the winter of 2021, I miss the sense of play and spontaneity. Despite how fortunate and grateful I know I am, I still struggle with how much the world has changed and become so divisive. And let's not forget how we all sort of went crazy too.

Remember when people were hoarding toilet paper and sanitized wipes? Then we moved on to collecting flour and yeast so we could bake bread and get fatter. I didn't need to watch the news to know that people lined up outside the grocery store, liquor store, dollar store, pharmacy. If you're not wearing a mask, you're denied entry whether you're picking up pizza or life-saving medicine. There are still plenty of days when I wish I could engage more with this brave new world that has emerged but there's still so much at stake should I get sick. I am looking forward to my life expanding beyond the boundaries of my home and backyard. Happily, those days are upon me, one step at a time.

Throughout 2020 and right to today, I am especially impressed by Lauren's sacrifices for me. I realize my health status shapes her choices. My daughter has chosen to follow my lead in not going anywhere or seeing anyone. Her rationale is that if she is out among the masses, there's a greater likelihood she can bring home a virus, whether a flu or COVID. I so appreciate her care and concern for me. I wish I were healthier and stronger. On bad days, there are times I resent feeling like a burden to my beautiful daughter who's in the prime of her life. I know I am not the only parent who feels this way. But Lauren continues to persevere. She's gone back to school and is working on her Masters in Education. She is regularly perched in front of a screen, learning and studying. Strange days. This new direction of hers has given us more motivation to get back to doing our H.O.G.: Hour of Goodness. What started off as a resolution at the beginning of 2020 has been reenergized and restarted. Each day we make time for writing (me) and studying (Lauren). You do what you do to make it through. For me and my daughter, an Hour of Goodness blesses us with strength and focus.

I will admit that my impressive motivation mindset (if I do say so myself) and regular sources of joy and inspiration often fail me. Getting things done takes more work these days. Trauma specialists tell us that during a trauma, such as a global pandemic, part of our brain shuts down so we're better able to survive. Me? I'd much rather thrive and I know you would too. The brain shutdown means we are not able to process a lot of what is going on around us. This leaves us feeling numb and out of touch with our emotions. Being kind to ourselves and taking care of each other, as much as we can, is so important. I'm saddened when I hear about the rising addiction and suicide numbers yet I'm eerily unsurprised. We are social and loving creatures. Humans are not meant to live apart from one another, especially apart from those we love the most.

I have heard it said that in times like this, when our focus in life has changed drastically, we are given the opportunity to learn life lessons. I am beginning to see that I need to learn how to be good to myself. Cut myself some slack, not be so hard on my weak spots or failings. I seem to have a habit of thinking that what I do or say is not good enough. I love me, but I'm hard on me. Lauren and I are trying to hold each other accountable in terms of self care and self talk (more positive, less negative). Living together full time gives both of us plenty of opportunity to give and receive reminders about commitments we've promised ourselves. You know, dreams and goals otherwise known as "get off the couch" or "go outside and get some fresh air" directives. With so much time at home and with each other, it's imperative we gain positive momentum as we build more positive routines. I consider our self-care focus a vital part of our re-entry training into the social world. And my, how the world has changed: sitting apart, never touching, and all of us wearing masks! Some days I don't know whether to laugh, cry or scream. I keep reminding myself, "This too shall pass." Easier said than done when the hours, days, and weeks are slipping by.

I know I am not the only one in the world who needs to be so careful, but it is hard not to spend some time feeling sorry for myself. Often I wake up in a funk and know that it is going to be tough to pull myself out of a dark place. Other times, I talk to someone about things they are doing and people they are seeing, and I can feel the "woe is me" wave coming. The little girlies, my granddaughters, are now spending more time with their other grandparents, which is wonderful for all of them, but it is hard not to feel envious. I am grateful for so much. We have a house that we are safe in. Lauren and I have each other. Shamus and April and the girls are close by, friends are caring and reaching out. We are really and truly blessed. My prayer is for a quick end to this strange way of living, but the reality is that we have no control over any of it.

What gets me through this crazy time is that when this pandemic is over (or at least controlled), I will be able to hug my granddaughters and the rest of my family. I will be able to get a haircut. Lauren and I will feel less isolated. My daughter will be able to meet with friends again and make new ones. Our lives will open and our smiles will brighten, which people will be able to see because we're not muzzled with masks. Wouldn't that be nice?

All these wishes passed through my mind as I blew out my 2020 birthday candles this July. I had arranged for the family to come for dinner. We'd ordered in, set up tables outside, and practised physical distancing. No hugs for this birthday girl! The forecast was for rain, which is unusual for my birthday since mid-July almost always brings warmth and sunshine. Of course, this year was different. What wasn't different? Lauren tidied up our garage and made space for us to eat, just in case the rain poured down. Perfect. In the morning, a friend came over, bringing tea and goodies. We visited for a couple of lovely hours in the garage. The rustic location fazed neither of us. I was with my friend, I was laughing, eating cookies, and feeling great.

Then it was nap time.

The family arrived around 5:00 that evening and more fun began. Cards, presents, and the gift of being together. The kids had ordered me a hammock. Nice. Perfect for the lazy summer days lying ahead. I was then presented with a giant overflowing gift bag. I had to follow step-by-step instructions. Before I knew it, I was covered in plastic. My entire body was "mummified" even my head and face, but of course I had a blow hole. (This wasn't a murderous birthday party!) There was great laughter and frivolity going on, yet I still had no idea what the gift was. The sound of my family's laughter was priceless and inspired my own giggles. Absolute silliness and an absolute delight. Who knew you could have so much fun inside a garage? The final detail was that I had my eyes masked. I joked that I was being kidnapped and put on Maid of the Mist boat in Niagara Falls.

As I stood there wrapped, rolled and blind, I became aware of someone getting close to me. But why? In a moment, Shamus had his big, strong arms around me. A hug. After four months of not being able to hug anyone but Lauren, there was my boy, hugging me. I was so overwhelmed with emotion that I could not even cry properly. For those few seconds it felt like my life was, once again, full and complete. Feeling complete is how I define the feeling of joy. I felt such gratitude for something so simple and pure, a hug. Love and wonderment made from plastic bags. Welcome to pandemic creativity!

Shamus and I held each other for so long. We drew apart hesitantly. He'd deny it but I think he was crying too. Then again, I was still blindfolded so what do I know? Next in line to give and receive hugs: Emma, Lily and their mother. April later modestly admitted that it was she who'd thought up how to bless me with safe and loving hugs. I could hear Lauren sniffling and laughing. And recording every second on her phone, I later discovered. Those hugs were the most amazing birthday gift I've ever received. I still glow from the impact of that loving circle. The pandemic has stolen much from each of us whether our losses are tiny or terrible. For me, my birthday in the summer of 2020 was a kind of reclamation. With those hugs, I was reassured we'd all make it through, each and everyone of us. It's a vision and a prayer I still hold in my heart today.

I know this pandemic will eventually end. "Just be patient," I keep saying to myself. "Be patient, impatient patient!" my inner self hollers and then laughs. I guess she knows, and wants us to know, things are turning out all right. We're getting through this terrible thing, together.

Chapter 23

Looking Back, Looking Forward

Which is better, looking back or looking forward? A memoir is, by definition, looking back at life. Given the way the world is at the moment, I think looking back helps us realize all that we have to be grateful for. Also, how challenges build courage, empathy, and resilience. Always remember how strong you can get when things do not go exactly as planned. No matter how tough and terrible life gets, we need to remember the lessons we have learned. When perceived freedoms are taken away, we quickly see and feel our sources of gratitude. For most of us, it's being able to spend time with those we love. Or appreciating the "luxury" of running to the store for a last-minute ingredient. Another big one for me, I admit, is being able to get my hair cut and feel pretty. I miss laughing and gossiping with my hairstylist. She's a gem, and I miss her. I miss life before the pandemic just as I miss life when I'm feeling sick and wishing I felt strong.

Gratitude has helped me through all of my difficulties in life. There are times when it's hard to feel grateful. When I was involved in my last relationship (which ended many years ago) there were times when it was hard to feel grateful. Another time when gratitude or perspective eluded me was when my brother Jay died. I felt so bereft. He and I were close and just like that, he was gone. I was as close to grateful as I could be when Mom died only because I knew she truly was in a better place.

Part of being human is feeling and thinking that gratitude is simply impossible. Life can be so hard and so cruel. The thing is, you do not have to look far to find people facing more pain or dealing with situations bordering on the catastrophic. Yet so much of what we complain about is more about inconvenience and impatience than the big and deadly stuff: loss of your health or loss of your loved one(s). Losing what you love makes you stronger and, I hope, kinder and more compassionate toward yourself and others. Life gets easier and richer, and is definitely infused with more gratitude and grace, when we understand that we're all dealing with issues the best way we can.

Over the years I've come to realize that one of my most emotionally difficult times happened while I was in a relationship that lasted longer than it should have. For years afterwards I could not see, much less feel, gratitude for the experience, which I judged as harmful to me and those I cherished the most. Looking back generally offers 20/20 vision yet I still wish (as likely you do) that there could be a little hint of where our lives are going when we're making plans and allowing people into our lives. Wouldn't it be nice if we had a sort of guidepost or map that would help us make empowered and informed decisions? Alas, there is no map, only our heart lines and frown lines. We do the best we can with the information we have at the time. So often a "gut feeling" has shaped my decisions. When I've trusted my intuition, I've made positive decisions. When I've ignored my intuition, you can imagine the outcome in general terms: pain and suffering alert! That failed relationship of mine was a classic example of not trusting my gut (or my brain!) and moving forward with the doomed, misplaced hope that a person or circumstance will change.

Nope.

Of course, once we have lived through a terrible experience, we eventually, hopefully and with intention and effort, come to see how things worked out for the best. Looking back on my last relationship, which, if you remember, dear reader, was with a man who graciously donated his kidney to me, I still ask myself a lot of questions about what unfolded: why did such negative things happen? Why was there so much pain inflicted on me and those around me? Why was a life-saving gift (his kidney) not enough to bond us together but instead tore us apart? My former partner and kidney donor approached life differently than I. He was opinionated and his thoughts and ideas were the right ones, and the only point of view that counted. Ever.

How do you like it so far? Yes, a match made in heaven, indeed.

Because of our conflicting worldviews (yes, I too am opinionated but I bend and sometimes too much and too often) there was so much conflict. I did my best to not argue with him. I didn't have the energy or the interest. There was a lot of miscommunication. Not really hearing each other. Of course, I think he didn't listen to me and I was probably just as guilty of hearing words but not listening mindfully. I consider myself a fair and flexible person, but I would still not list "tolerance and flexibility" as Ernest's strongest qualities.

In retrospect, what I see when I think of Ernest is a kidney donor who had very little experience with medical issues and was slightly afraid of the entire transplantation process. His bravado didn't serve him well. For example, he brought a bag of books to the hospital, assuming he would bounce back immediately after surgery. The severity of the surgery had been explained to him. I mean, donating a kidney is major surgery. Again, maybe he didn't listen? Didn't want to know? All couples have ups and downs. Imagine feeling that your partner has inflicted physical pain on you for their own physical benefit. Imagine feeling your partner is resentful of you because he's been temporarily weakened as you grow in strength and vitality?

Yes, a kidney match made in heaven that delivered us straight to miscommunication hell for five years. There is humour in this story. Like, where we met. God sent an angel to heal me and my dying kidney. And where did that angel called Ernest appear? At church, of course. If I could speak to the younger self I once was, I would say, "Melody, you need to know and believe in yourself. Good job on working to make the relationship survive. Also, good job being understanding of his differences, of his opinions, and his way of life. And nice job providing for Ernest financially even though supporting him was a strain."

But my pep talk to my younger self wouldn't stop there. There are always at least two sides to a story, so I'd offer up a couple of "growth opportunities" to the woman I was back then when I was getting my second transplant. To the younger but not wiser Melody, I'd say, "Because I love you so much, here are three things you're doing very, very wrong. These three things are going to cost you for quite some time. First and foremost, you should have stood up to him against his verbal abuse of Lauren. Number two, you should not have let him bully you, even though he was taking care of you. You deserve to be cherished, then and now. Last and not least, younger Melody, your third big mistake or growth opportunity you need to learn from? You were so busy feeling desperate for a kidney that you put up with all this bad behaviour instead of trusting in me (God, spirit, the universe, however you like it). Melody, you always would have been provided for and strengthened. You didn't have to sacrifice so much."

Oh, the joys of 20/20 vision in 2020. So much time to stare at the wall and think about the past.

No one will ever take advantage of me, or my family, like Ernest did ever again. I have become much more independent and have learned to stand up for myself. Until our relationship dissolved, I had never been on my own, without a man in my life. Life is very manageable and much calmer without a man on the scene, I've discovered. For that pearl of hard-earned wisdom, I am grateful.

Once we have looked back and realized what we have had and may have lost, we are better able to look forward. By looking back, I more easily and joyfully can envision a positive and joyful future. Events I am looking forward to including finishing this memoir. The writing has been a long, hard process but so worthwhile. I certainly look forward to being able to spend time with the rest of my family and my friends without physical distancing or masks. I look forward to sitting in my backyard and hosting a BBQ or calling up a girlfriend and meeting her for lunch or tea. When I imagine the future, I see a future without limitation and without restrictions. As I bet you do! Of course, time will tell what the future holds. Looking forward, at best, is speculation.

We have seen that even though we may make plans, those plans may get turned upside down in a short period of time. The thing about making decisions is to remember that you need to remain flexible and willing to change. The thing about being flexible is that you never know when challenges will arise. For instance, last Sunday after dinner, I began to feel unwell yet again. I went to bed and watched as my temperature rose and my tummy grew more and more bloated. Lauren insisted I go to hospital and I was equally adamant that I stay home. At one point I even told her to stop harassing me. Yet I knew in my heart of hearts that my daughter's concern was valid: I was sick and my condition was worsening. I was unsteady on my feet and burning with fever. I do not enjoy being in hospital at the best of times and during a pandemic is hardly "the best of times."

Lauren persevered and called Shamus to drive me, once again, to Emergency. I had been away from the hospital for less than a month. Again, when you're sick your quality of life is diminished so quickly and cruelly. The kids had packed up all my electronics and their chargers, my toothbrush, and hairbrush. Shamus and Lauren knew the drill. My overnight bag was a tangible and undeniable sign that I was going to be admitted to hospital for an indefinite amount of time. Oh, and don't forget the deadly pandemic virus that absolutely adored targeting older, immune-compromised, sick people trapped in overcrowded hospitals! If that car ride to ER had a theme? "Woe is me" and "Why me?" and "Why now?"

After more than 36 years, Tim's beautiful kidney, his gift to me, was kicking up a fuss. My first transplanted kidney was infected. There was some talk about removing the kidney, which did not seem like a good idea to me considering surgery would extend my time in hospital. Later that night at about 3 a.m. I wanted a cup of tea to soothe my nerves, spirit, and maybe even my poor kidney. One of the nurses managed to find a tea bag, heat up some water in the microwave, and bring me the concoction in a paper cup. The tea was awful, possibly the worst tea I've ever tasted. I searched for gratitude in my imaginary tea leaves but found none.

The morning's parade of doctors was impressive. There was the regular doctor (the "medicine doctor" is my nickname) who did rounds and oversaw all the patients. He poked and prodded me. Then came the infectious diseases doctor followed by the nephrologist (kidney specialist), and eventually the GI (gastrointestinal) doctor. These were all nice people, certainly looking out for my best interests. Was my dream team of doctors successful in restoring me to health and keeping Tim's kidney with me? Indeed they were. Was I sad when I left their hospital and returned home? No.

It's hard to believe that as the pandemic winds down, my health is looking up. Who would believe that coming out of a pandemic I would be stronger than I have been for years? As I heal, the world is also healing. Just as the pandemic is brought under control, my book writing is drawing to a close at last, at last. The pandemic has forced all of us to look back and look within. Today we are finally beginning to look toward the future with a kind of fragile hope and faith. Or at least I am. As always, the gift of gratitude continues to sustain me. Lily told me the other day that I had too many friends. I do have more friends visiting me now whether in the garage or in the backyard. I enjoy the social interactions, the infrequent, once-forbidden hugs. I am constantly seeing and believing that people care about me.

Even with all that I have been through, and certainly in light of what has happened these past 18 months, I am still continually shown how beautiful and fragile life is. We need to truly seize the day and make the most of our lives, come what may. This may be the end of my memoir, but I will never be done with life. Or with my love for you. And you. And you. And you. I am grateful to have loved so many and been loved by so many, deeply and as myself.

I could have asked for an easier life, but I could not have asked for a better life. I've been given two gifts during this lifetime. Both were gifts of life manifesting as healthy kidneys, offering well-being, health, and vitality. But the joy in my life has always come from my family, my children, and my friends. I am grateful for this life and your role in my wild and wonderful adventure.

Forever Grateful

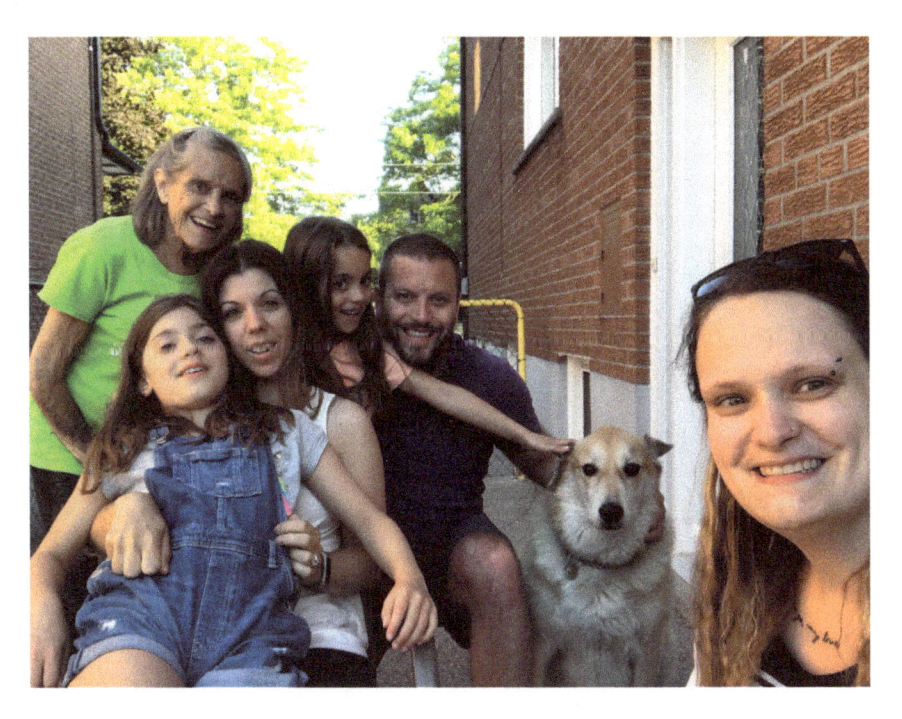

My wonderful family, summer 2021
(L to R) Me, Emma, April, Lily, Shamus, Koda, Lauren

Acknowledgements

There are so many people I want to acknowledge. Without them this book may not have come to fruition. First and foremost, I am grateful to my parents, Ina and Wesley Klassen. Mom and Dad were always supportive, understanding, and encouraging. They were both gone before I began this endeavour but if they'd been here, they'd have cheered on this giant undertaking. My parents were always my biggest cheering section.

My brothers, David, Tim, and Jay. There are not enough words to express my love and gratitude for my brother Tim. Tim, thank you. You selflessly gave of yourself so I could have a better life, a life better than I could have ever imagined. To Ernest, my second donor: thank you for helping me and giving me back my health and freedom to live without dialysis.

The Canadian healthcare system has been a godsend to me. When I think about the amount of healthcare I have received over the years and how that life-saving care has cost nothing out of my own wallet (except taxes), I am overcome with gratitude. Thank you, Tommy Douglas.

I definitely want to acknowledge the special men who played such an important role in realizing one of my lifelong dreams: becoming a mother. Thank you, Adrian and Bob. Without you I would not have our two precious children, Shamus and Lauren.

There is a whole list of doctors and medical professionals who've been instrumental in the hard work of keeping me healthy, happy, and alive. My heartfelt thanks to my "kidney team": Dr. M. McCann (my GP who originally diagnosed kidney disease), Dr. D. Cattran (my first nephrologist at Toronto General Hospital), Brenda McQuarrie (Transplant Coordinator at Toronto General), and Dr. J. Zaltzman (nephrologist at St. Michael's Hospital). Special thanks also go out to Dr. Shear (dermatologist), Dr. Grover (Gastrointestinal), and Dr. JC Monge (cardiologist). These wonderful doctors have acted like medical detectives in their attempts to solve and lessen the impact of certain medications on me.

I want to especially acknowledge my children, the first real loves of my life. They are wonderful human beings and they keep me grounded. It has been such a joy to watch them grow and develop into the people they are now. I cannot even imagine what life would have been like if they had never come into my life.

Shamus, watching you as a husband and parent is incredible. Your love and compassion for the ladies in your life is wonderful. I include myself as one of those ladies. You are a good son, a loving brother, husband, and dad. I am so proud of you.

Lauren, I am so blessed to have you as my companion, especially over the last year. Without you life would have been close to unbearable. Your love of children, animals, and music is thrilling. Never lose your passion for any of them. You are a delight and a sweetheart, and so strong. I believe in you always.

Then there are my precious grandchildren, my girlies: Emma and Lily. You bring such joy and delight to my life. You are sunshine to everyone in your orbit. I love you both with all my heart, and Granny's heart is big! Emma, continue to use your smarts and your sense of humour. You will always be my sunshine. Lily, you are such a dear soul and I suspect an old soul. Your delightful wit is emotional and passionate. You have wisdom beyond your years.

I have been blessed with so many good and loving friends. They continue to support and encourage me. Some have been friends for many, many years and some are newer in my life, but you have all added so much. To my friends, there are so many. Ruth, Beth, Diane, Diana,

Andra, Pat (there seem to be many Pats in my life!), Katharine, Linda, Ana, Beth, Carole, Donna, Heather, Janet, Meg, Jason, Lynn, Paulette. I am so blessed. If you're not on this list, it's because you're shy and I didn't want to make you blush! All kidding aside, my life would lack colour without my friendships. You know who you are. Please know your love and care continually amaze me. I am grateful you are part of my life.

A special shout-out to Shannon Leahy. I could not have ever dreamed of finishing this work of love if it had not been for your support and encouragement. Shannon, you have been a true leading light in my writing journey. Continue to shine on, my dear friend.

My life has been challenging in lots of ways but without you, the people I love and cherish, my adventure here would not have been nearly as interesting or as filled with love. I am blessed with miracles and gratitude in my life. Thank you for reading my tall melodious tales.

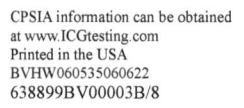

CPSIA information can be obtained
at www.ICGtesting.com
Printed in the USA
BVHW060535060622
638899BV00003B/8